# simply
# healthy food

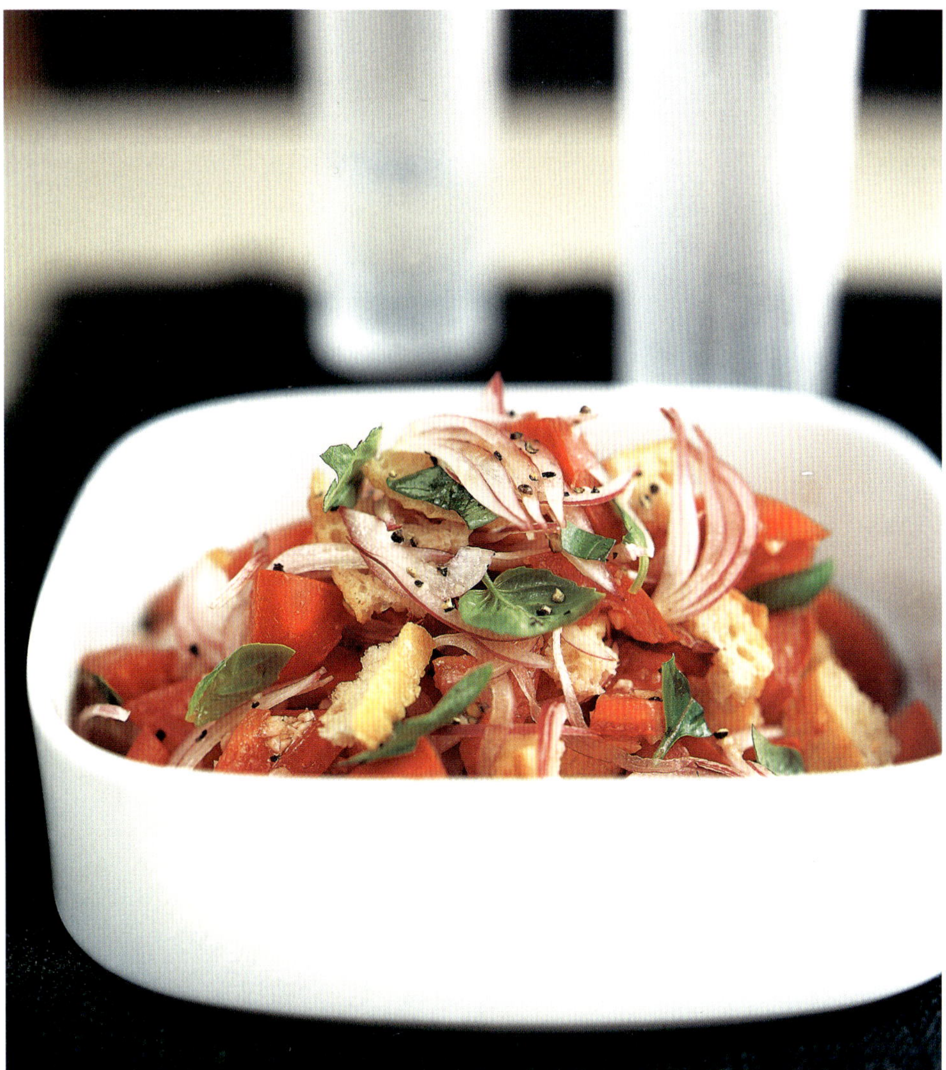

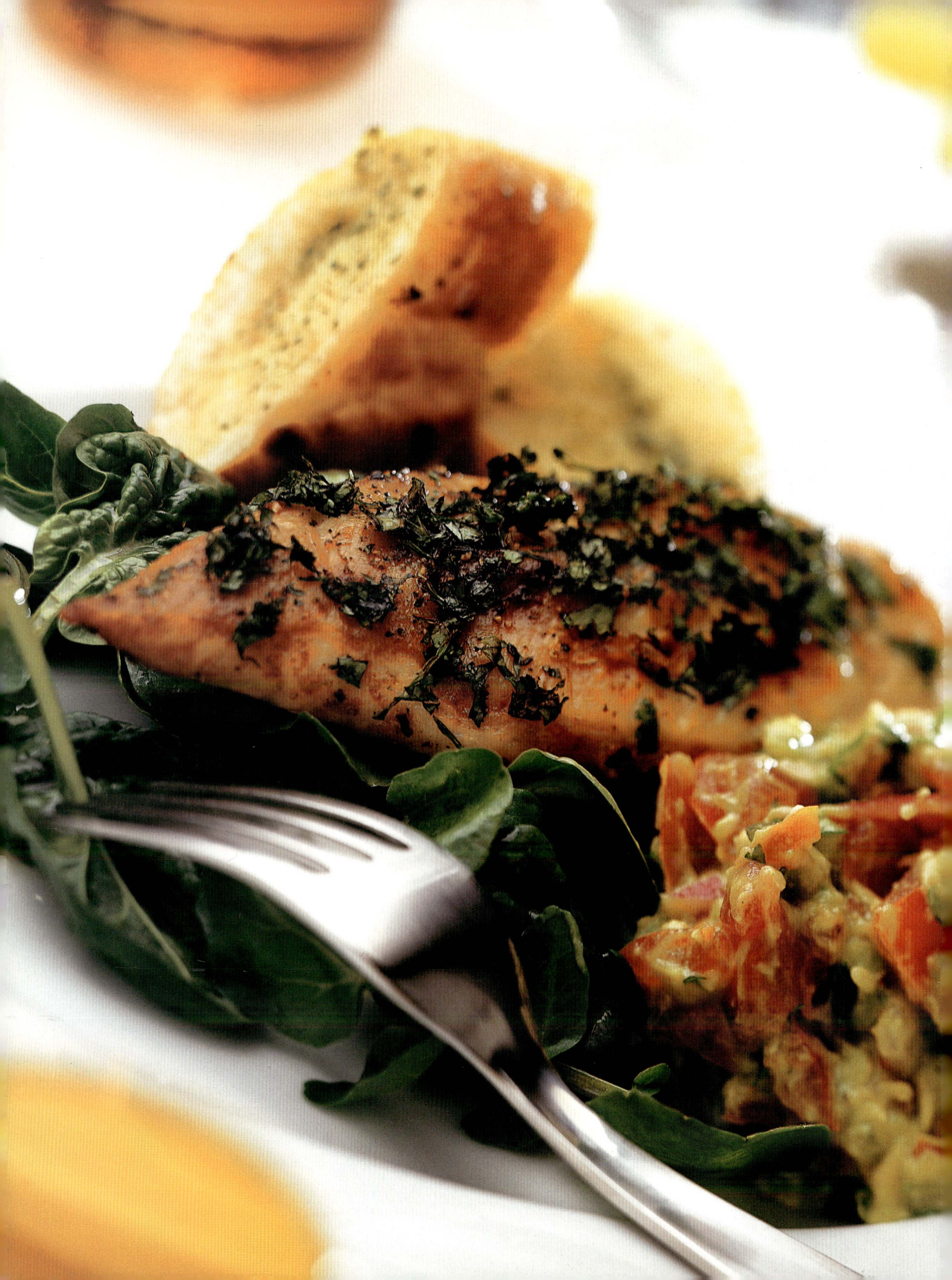

# simply
# healthy food

over **175 recipes and ideas** for food that does you good

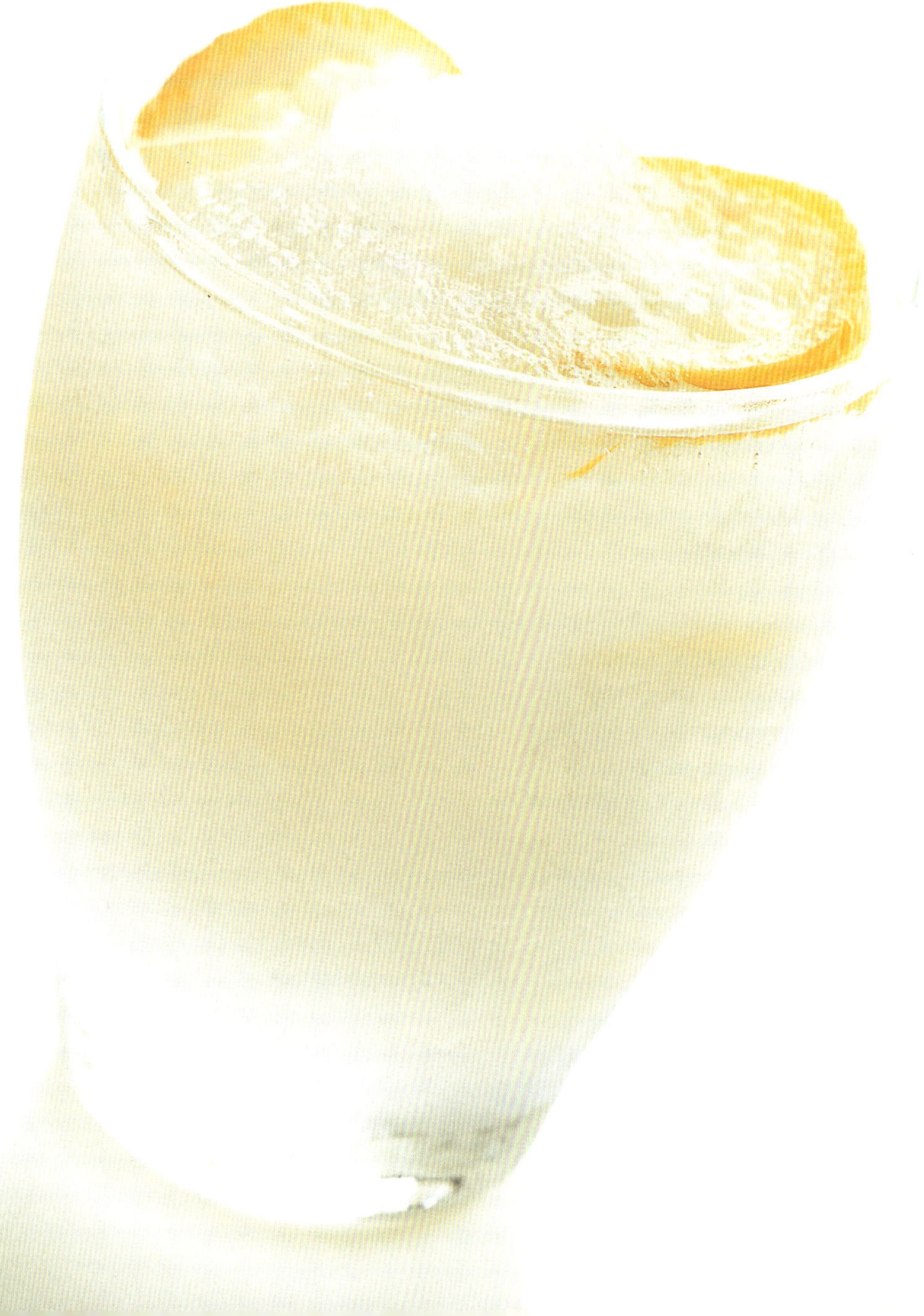

quadrille

First published in 2002 by
**Quadrille Publishing Limited**
Alhambra House
27–31 Charing Cross Road
London WC2H OLS

The material in this volume was previously published
in *BBC Good Food* magazine.



ISBN 1 903845 21 1

Editor & Project Manager: **Lewis Esson**
Editorial Director: **Jane O'Shea**
Creative Director: **Mary Evans**
Art Director: **Helen Lewis**
Design Assistant: **Katy Davis**
Project Editor for the BBC: **Vicki Vrint**
Production: **Nancy Roberts**

Printed and bound in Singapore.

- Throughout the book recipes are for four people unless otherwise stated.
- Both metric and imperial quantities are given. Use either all metric or all imperial, as the two are not necessarily interchangeable.

# Contents

# Introduction

*The message of this book is that healthy eating needn't mean dull food or missing out on all the things that you love. Balance and variety have always been the watchwords of a good diet, and recent discoveries have shown this to be even wiser advice than we ever thought.*

*As well as the essential vitamins and minerals, scientists have lately discovered that many foods - particularly plant-based produce, like fruit, vegetables, pulses, seeds and grains - contain a wide range of phytochemicals that actively help to prevent and/or fight serious life-threatening conditions like cancer and heart disease. So the wider a range of foods we eat, particularly if we favour fruit and vegetables, the more we benefit from this extraordinary natural medicine chest - hence the whole emphasis on the 'superfoods' and getting our 'five-a-day'.*

*In Simply Healthy Food, we have collected together a variety of recipes for tasty and exciting dishes that will help you make the most of this bounty. Each is selected to provide healthy levels of the major nutrients, like protein, fat, cholesterol and fibre, and wherever possible at least one of these 'superfoods', packed full of protective power.*

*You'll also find some very surprising foods featured in the book, like eggs and chocolate, and you'll learn that these are not the demons that they have been made out to be, but that it is the saturated fat - and sugar in the latter case - that often come along with them that are the problems. You'll also discover that, although it's generally advisable to cut down on the amount of fat (and sugar and salt) in our diets, some fats are actually 'superfoods' - like olive oil and the omega-3s in oily fish.*

*The simple aim of this book is to help readers see that healthy eating can be an exciting voyage of discovery, not a prison of dietary constraints. In fact, our real definition of 'good food' is 'food that does you good'.*

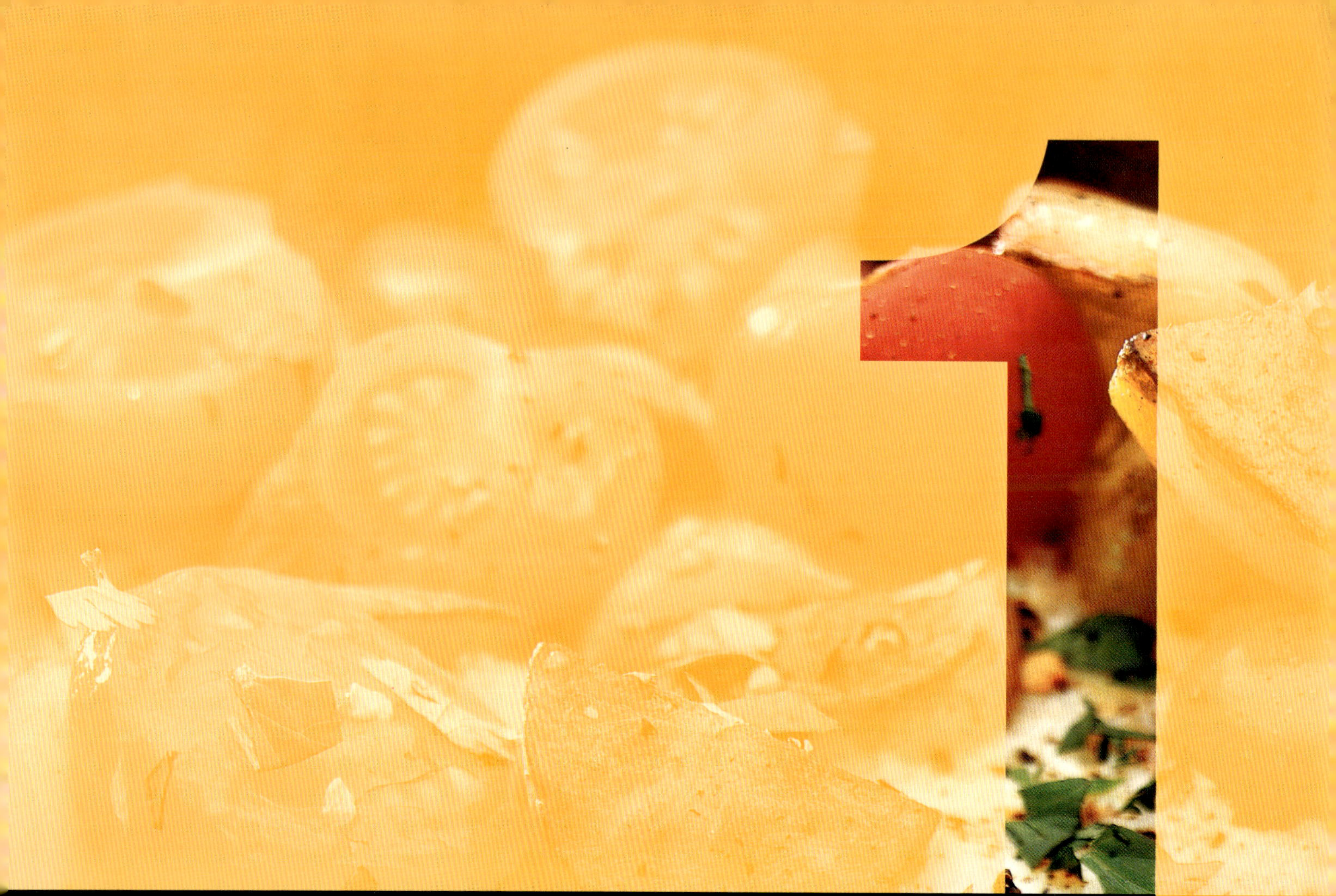

1

# Blooming Breakfasts and Lunches

*The old adage that one should 'breakfast like a king and dine like a pauper' couldn't better express a plan for healthy eating. As well as providing you with energy for the day ahead, a good balanced breakfast gives you a chance to start the day with a valuable proportion of your vitamin and mineral requirements. It will also probably mean that you will be less likely to indulge in sugary snacks and that the rest of your eating during the day will also be more balanced.*

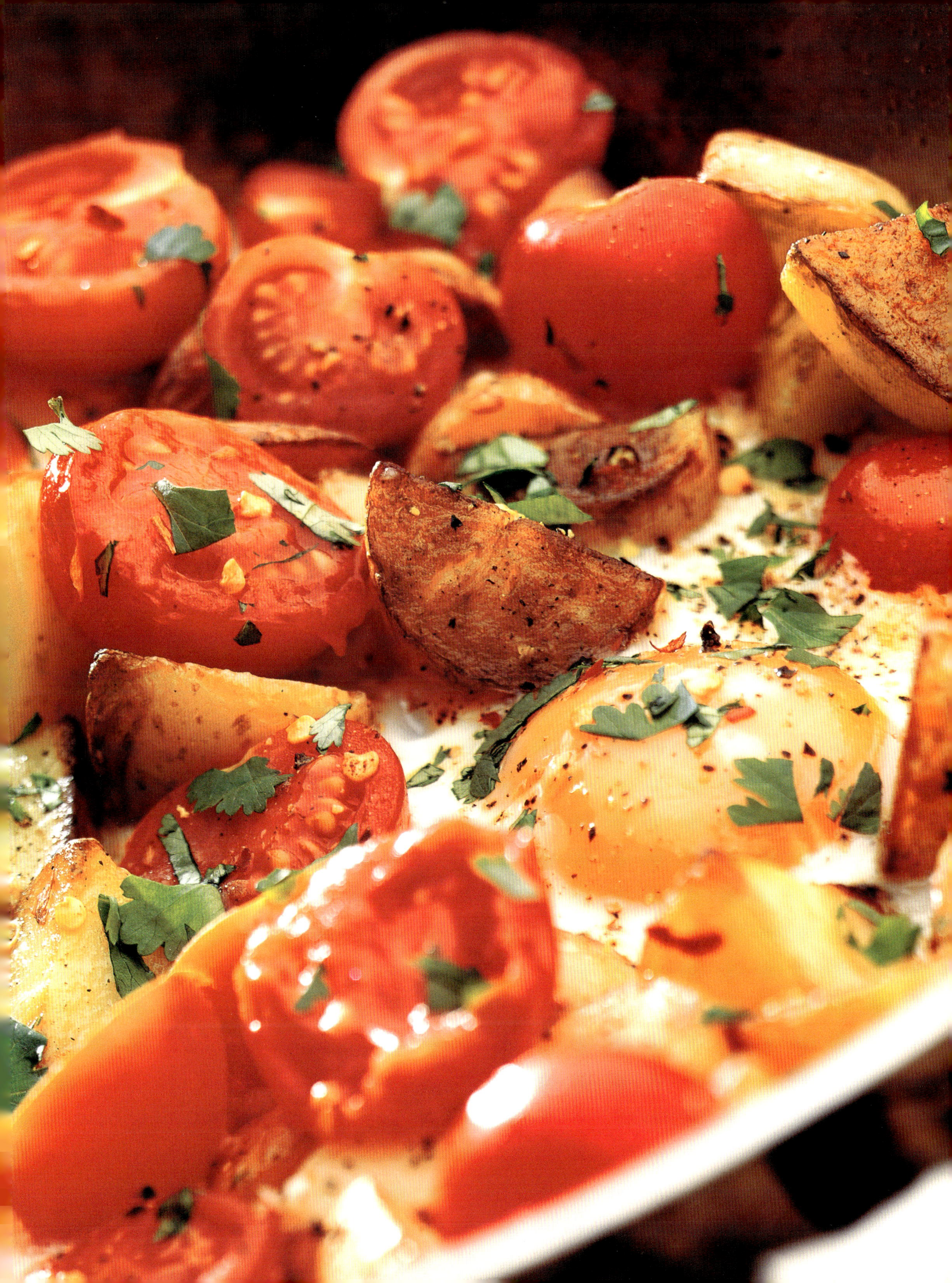

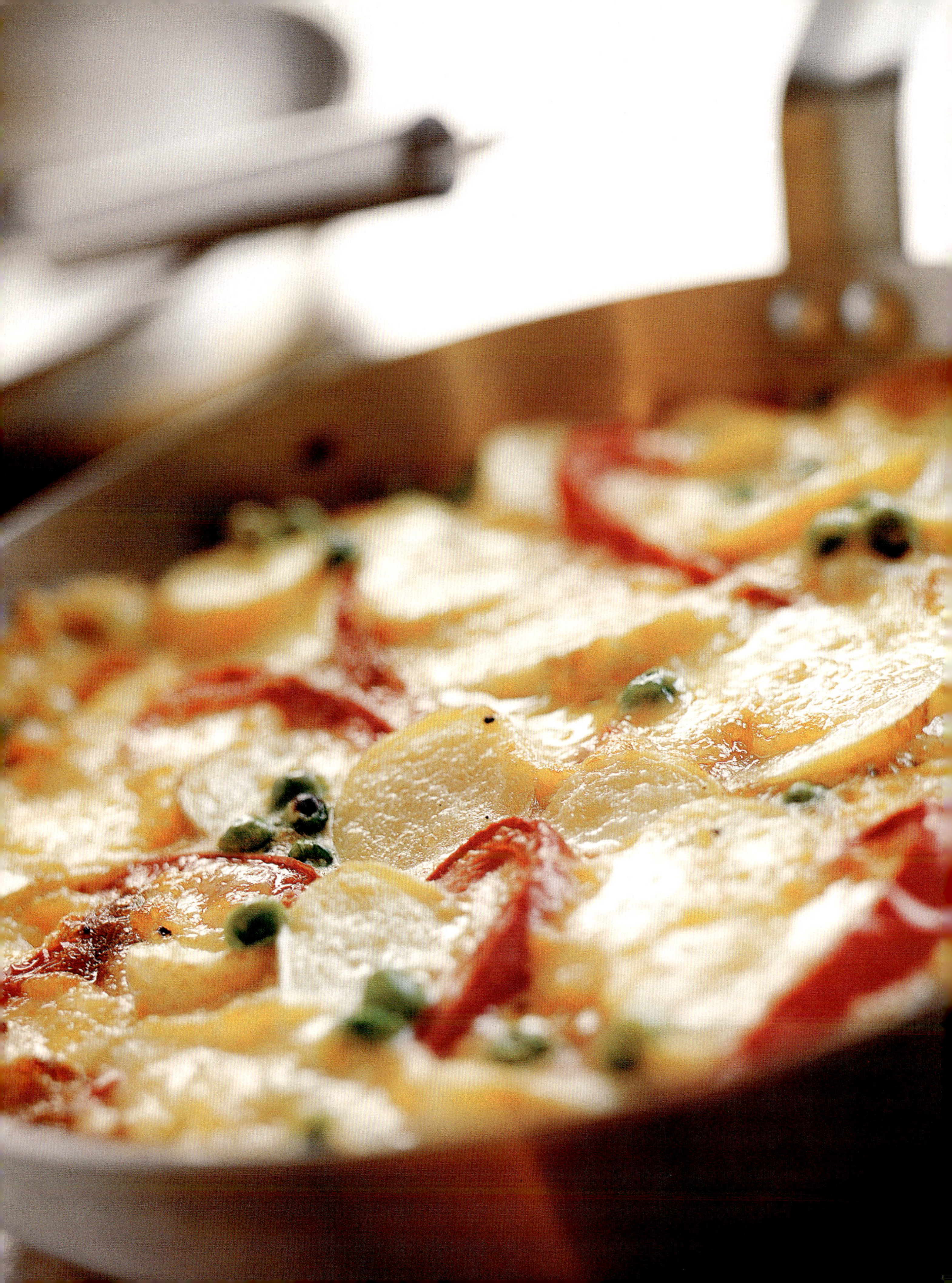

# Eggs from the Med

PER SERVING
458 kcalories
protein 19g
carbohydrate 47g
fat 23g
saturated fat 5g
fibre 4g
added sugar none
salt 0.71g

**Surprise, surprise... eggs fried in a little vegetable or olive oil do actually help make a healthy breakfast, providing just enough fat and protein to keep hunger pangs at bay for the rest of the morning. The potatoes help ensure that your blood sugar levels stay on a fairly even keel and the tomatoes go towards your five fruit and veg a day. Eggs also provide you with vitamins B12, A and D, folate and iodine and, to a lesser extent, B2, E and nicotinic acid. Eggs are, of course, high in cholesterol, but this is usually not a problem unless your diet is overly high in saturated fats (see page 94).**

SERVES 2
PREPARATION about 15 minutes
COOKING about 20 minutes

2 tbsp olive oil
500g/1lb 2oz new potatoes, cut into small chunks
3 pinches of chilli flakes or powder
1 garlic clove, chopped
225g/8oz small tomatoes, halved
4 eggs
a good handful of roughly chopped coriander leaves

1 Heat the olive oil in a large, preferably non-stick, pan. Add the potatoes and fry over a high heat until they start to colour, then sprinkle in the chilli flakes or powder, garlic and salt and pepper to taste. Cover and cook for about 10 minutes until the potatoes are just tender.
2 Throw in the tomatoes and cook for a few minutes until they start to soften.
3 Make 4 gaps in the mixture, then break an egg into each one. Season, then cover and cook for 3–4 minutes until the eggs are softly set (or to your liking).
4 Scatter over the chopped coriander leaves and serve straight from the pan.

# Potato and Red Pepper Tortilla

PER SERVING
352 kcalories
protein 19g
carbohydrate 23g
fat 21g
saturated fat 7g
fibre 3g
added sugar none
salt 0.86g

**Frozen peas are almost more nutritious than fresh – packed with a wide range of vitamins and minerals – as they are usually frozen so promptly after harvesting.**

PREPARATION about 15 minutes
COOKING about 30 minutes

450g/1lb new potatoes, cut into thin slices
2 tbsp olive oil
1 red pepper, deseeded and sliced
100g/4oz frozen peas
6 eggs
60g/2oz mature Cheddar cheese

1 Cook the potatoes in a pan of lightly salted boiling water for about 10 minutes, until almost tender. Drain well, then return the potatoes to the pan to dry.
2 Heat the oil in a large frying pan, add the pepper and fry for 2–3 minutes until softened. Add the potatoes and cook for 3–4 minutes until lightly browned, then throw in the peas.
3 Beat the eggs in a bowl with a little salt and pepper and pour into the pan. Cook over a moderate heat for 8–10 minutes, until the tortilla is set on the bottom and sides and nearly firm in the middle. While the eggs are cooking, preheat the grill.
4 Cut or break the cheese into cubes and sprinkle over the tortilla. Put the pan under the preheated grill until the cheese has melted and is lightly browned.
5 Cut the tortilla into wedges and serve straight from the pan. Leftovers are great cold for picnics.

# Parsnip Pancakes with Soy Dipping Sauce

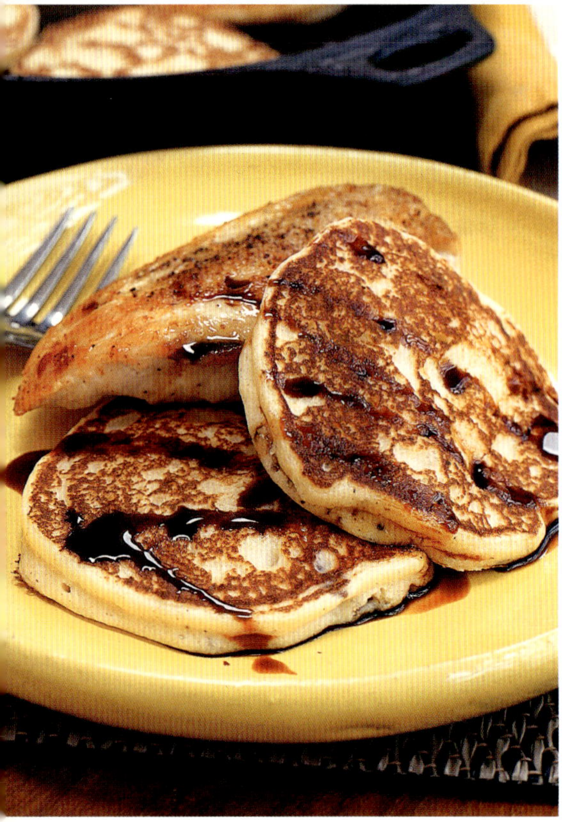

**A good source of fibre, parsnips also provide vitamins B1 and C, beta-carotene, nicotinic acid, folate, potassium, phosphorus and iron.**

**MAKES** 6
**PREPARATION** 30 minutes
**COOKING** 12 minutes

1 large parsnip, about 250g/9oz, peeled and cut into chunks
85g/3oz self-raising flour
1 egg, plus white of 1 more egg
150ml/¼ pint milk
large pinch of sugar, to taste
large knob of butter
soy sauce, for drizzling (optional)

**PER PANCAKE**
**120 kcalories • protein 4g • carbohydrate 18g fat 4g • saturated fat 2g • fibre 2g added sugar 1g • salt 1.17g**

1 Boil the parsnip in salted water for 15 minutes until soft. Drain and blend in a food processor until smooth.
2 Put the flour in a bowl and stir in the whole egg and parsnip purée. Gradually stir in milk to make a thick batter. Season and add the sugar.
3 In another bowl, whisk the egg white to soft peaks. Stir a third of it into the parsnip mix to slacken it, then carefully fold in the rest.
4 Heat half the butter in a large frying pan. When foaming, drop in 3 large spoonfuls (about a 3-tablespoon measure for each pancake) of batter. Cook for 3 minutes until the underside is golden and bubbles appear on top. Cook the other side until golden. Cook remaining pancakes similarly.
5 Serve drizzled with a splash of soy sauce if you like.

# Sweetcorn Fritters

**PER FRITTER**
**128 kcalories**
**protein 1g**
**carbohydrate 7g**
**fat 11g**
**saturated fat 2g**
**fibre 0.5g**
**added sugar none**
**salt 0.04g**

**If you grow sweetcorn, you'll know that - rushed from plant to pan - there is no vegetable more heavenly. Bought cobs never have quite the bouquet (the sugars start to turn to starch within two hours of picking). These fritters really make the most of sweetcorn, delivering lots of beta-carotene, folate, vitamin C and fibre. You can, of course, use 350g/12 oz frozen sweetcorn kernels instead.**

**MAKES** 12
**PREPARATION** 5 minutes
**COOKING** 15 minutes

3 fresh sweetcorn cobs
sunflower oil, for frying
4 tbsp extra-thick double cream or full-fat crème fraîche
2 tbsp self-raising flour

1 In a pan of boiling salted water, cook the corn cobs for 7–8 minutes. Remove from the heat and drain. When cool enough to handle, slice the kernels from the cob with a sharp knife.
2 Heat a little oil in a large non-stick frying pan until just smoking. Meanwhile, put the kernels in a bowl. Mix in the cream or crème fraîche, followed by the flour. Season.
3 Drop 4 spoonfuls of mixture into the oil. Flatten gently with a spatula (they will look slightly lacy) and fry for 3 minutes on each side until golden. (They are fragile, so use 2 spatulas to turn them.) Stand to one side, as they will pop a bit. Carefully remove the fritters, drain on kitchen paper and repeat the process until you have made 12.

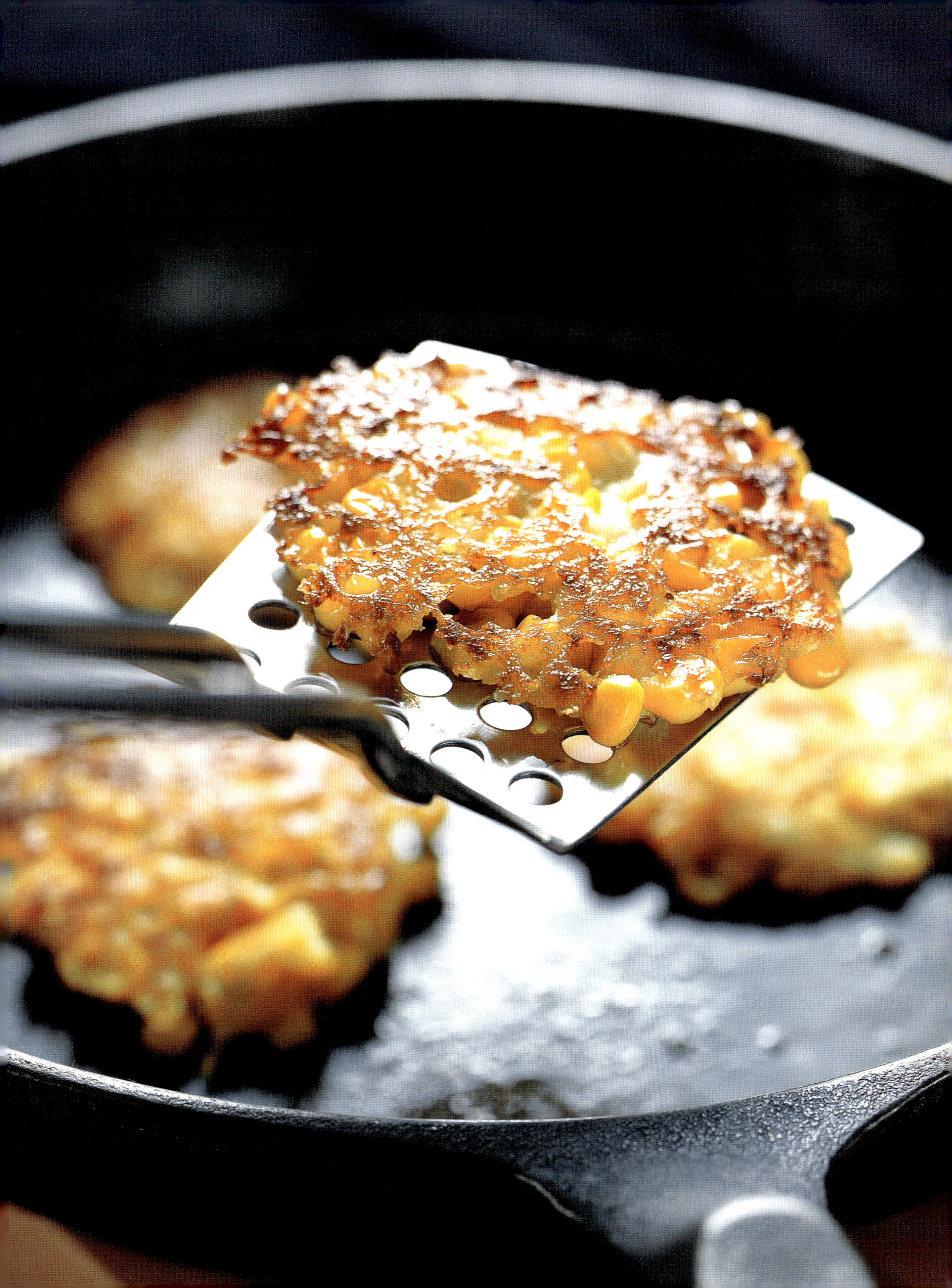

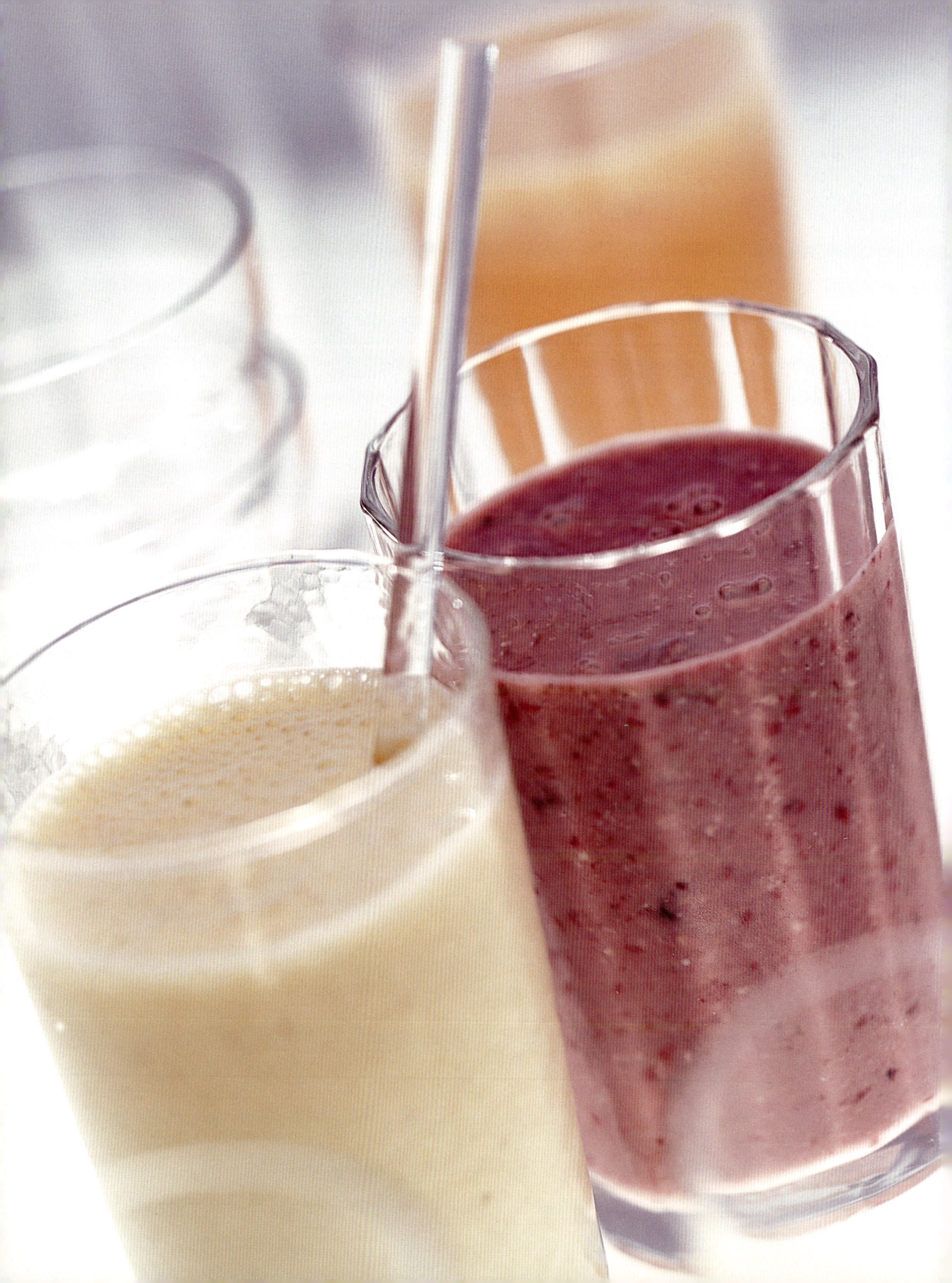

# Sensational Smoothies

**Smoothies are among the best of all possible ways to get a good, quick, super-healthy dose of fruit in the morning. Mixtures of coarsely chopped raw fruit with fruit juices and/or low-fat natural yoghurt are blitzed in a blender until fairly smooth. Using ready frozen fruit, or freezing the fruit ahead of time, chills the smoothie sufficiently without necessarily adding any ice, which can dilute the texture.**

EACH SERVES 2
PREPARATION 10 minutes

**for the sparkling tropical smoothie**

1 cup of orange juice
1 cup of chopped pineapple
chopped flesh of 1 ripe mango
ice
sparkling water

PER SERVING
**153 kcalories**
**protein 1.8g**
**carbohydrate 37.6g**
**fat 0.6g**
**saturated fat 0g**
**fibre 4.6g**
**added sugar 0g**
**salt 0g**

**for the berry oat smoothie**

2 tablespoons frozen chopped banana
1 cup of frozen raspberries, blackberries or blueberries (or a mixture)
2 tablespoons porridge oats
2 tablespoons runny low-fat natural yoghurt
300ml/ 1/2 pint apple juice

PER SERVING
**155 kcalories**
**protein 3.7g**
**carbohydrate 33.1g**
**fat 1.9g**
**saturated fat 0.4g**
**fibre 2.8g**
**added sugar 0g**
**salt 0g**

**for the pear, melon and cherry smoothie**

1 pear, peeled, cored and chopped
1 large cup of chopped orange-fleshed melon
3 tablespoons frozen cherries

PER SERVING
**59 kcalories**
**protein 0.8g**
**carbohydrate 14.2g**
**fat 0.2g**
**saturated fat 0g**
**fibre 2.3g**
**added sugar 0g**
**salt 0g**

1 To make the sparkling tropical smoothie: put the orange juice, chopped pineapple and mango in a blender and blitz until smooth. Then divide the mixture between 2 tall glasses. Add ice and top up with sparkling water.

2 To make the berry oat smoothie: put the frozen chopped banana, frozen berries, porridge oats, yoghurt and apple juice in a blender and blitz until smooth. Then divide the mixture between 2 tall glasses.

3 To make the pear, melon and cherry smoothie: put the chopped pear, melon and frozen cherries in a blender and blitz until smooth. Then divide the mixture between 2 tall glasses.

VARIATIONS

All sorts of fruits and other ingredients can be use to great effect in smoothies. Try apples with chopped fresh mint and lime juice; carrots with a lump of fresh root ginger and some orange juice; any mixture of red berries, apple or orange juice and yoghurt; pears, apples, nectarines and grapes with orange juice.

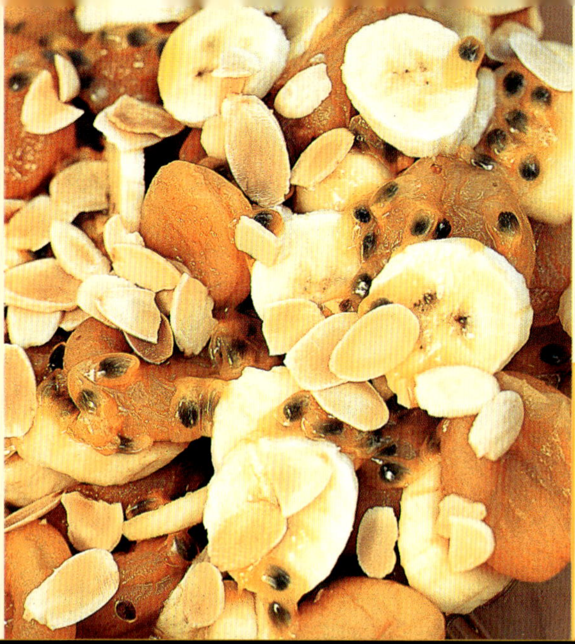

**PER SERVING**
**341 kcalories**
**protein 7g**
**carbohydrate 71g**
**fat 5g**
**saturated fat trace**
**fibre 8g**
**added sugar none**
**salt 0.13g**

# What is all this about 'five a day'?

*These days everyone is always talking about making sure you get your 'five a day' fruit and vegetables to ensure good health, but few sources actually ever give you more detail.*

**Why five?**

*Five portions of fruit and vegetables (about 400g/14oz in total) is the MINIMUM recommended by the world's health authorities. If you can fit more into your diet then all the better. Both fruit and vegetables are generally low in all the things that can be problematic and need careful monitoring and limiting – like fat, cholesterol and salt – while being rich in all other types of nutrients that are almost impossible to overdo. They are also sources of the recently discovered phytochemicals ('phyto' means 'from plants') that help the body actively fight off diseases ranging from colds and 'flus to cancers and heart disease.*

**What exactly constitutes a portion of fruit or veg?**

*It is fairly straightforward, at about 100g/4 oz uncooked weight per portion, with the exception of dried fruit, about 25g/¾ oz of which makes up a portion (as it is usually relatively high in sugar, it should also not really form more than one of your five a day). Generally, 1 orange, apple or banana constitutes a portion, as do 2 plums or kiwis, and a good large bowl of salad or about 150 ml/¼ pint of (pure and ideally freshly squeezed) fruit or vegetable juice. As juices contain little of the plant's natural fibre, they also should not form more than one of your five. It doesn't really matter if they have been cooked, as long as they don't have too much added fat, salt, etc., but it is better to ensure that at least one of your five a day is eaten raw.*

**Do all fruit and vegetables count?**

*Although a valuable part of your daily carbohydrate intake, starchy carbohydrates, like potatoes, sweet potatoes and yams, really should not be counted in your five a day, but most other root veg can. Also nuts and seeds, again although nutritionally important, don't count.*

**Is there a golden rule to 'five a day'?**

*Yes, variety... Try to build as wide a range of fruit and veg into your diet as you can. It's not really a good idea just to have the same things five times a day or every day as each plant has its own nutritional profile. This will ensure that you get a balance of the wonderful nutrients that the plant kingdom has to offer.*

**Breakfasts offer an excellent opportunity to get ahead on your five a day score ▶**

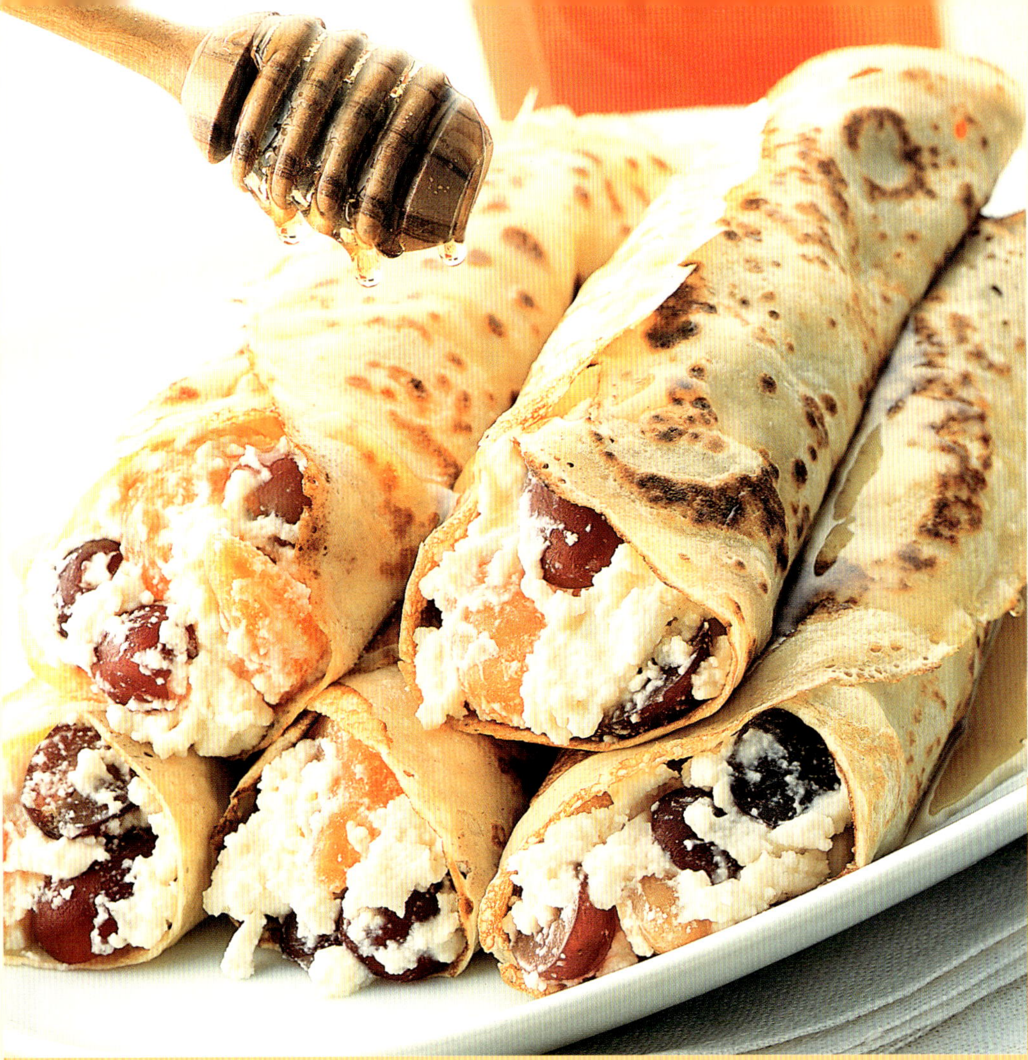

**PER PANCAKE**
**248 kcalories**
**protein 10g**
**carbohydrate 29g**
**fat 11g**
**saturated fat 6g**
**fibre 1g**
**added sugar 10g**
**salt 0.24g**

## Banana and Apricot Compote

*(opposite), for example, with a glass of fresh fruit juice, will get you over halfway there. Put 250g/9oz ready-to-eat dried apricots, 200ml/7fl oz apple juice (about a tumblerful) and 200ml/7fl oz water in a pan. Bring to the boil, cover and simmer for 20 minutes. Remove from the heat and leave to cool – you can make ahead up to this stage.*

*Tip the cooled apricots into a bowl and stir in 2 sliced bananas. Mix in the flesh from 4 passion fruits or a punnet of raspberries. Sprinkle 2 tablespoons toasted flaked almonds over the fruit and serve with yoghurt or crème fraîche, and your favourite biscuits.*

## Pancakes with Honey and Ricotta

*(above) as a breakfast treat allow you to change the fruits with the seasons. First make 8 pancakes: sift 100g/4oz plain flour into a bowl with a pinch of salt. Make a well in the centre of the flour, break in 1 egg and add about 3 tablespoons from 300ml/½ pint milk. Beat, gradually pouring in the rest of milk and drawing in the flour to make a smooth batter. Beat in 1 tablespoon sunflower oil or melted butter. The mixture should now resemble thin cream. (Alternatively, blend everything in a food processor for about 1½ minutes until smooth.)*

*Brush a pancake pan with oil or melted butter. When hot, add half a ladleful of the batter and quickly swirl the pan to coat it in a thin even layer. After about 1 minute, flip the pancake and cook the other side for about 30 seconds until brown. Remove and keep warm. Repeat with the remaining batter, wiping the pan with a little oil or butter between each pancake.*

*Mix two 250g/9oz tubs of ricotta or mascarpone with 4 tablespoons clear honey, then stir in 4 peeled, segmented and halved satsumas or mandarins, and 225g/8oz halved red grapes. Spoon the mixture down the centre of each pancake, then roll up like a cigar. Serve the stuffed pancakes drizzled with a little more honey.*

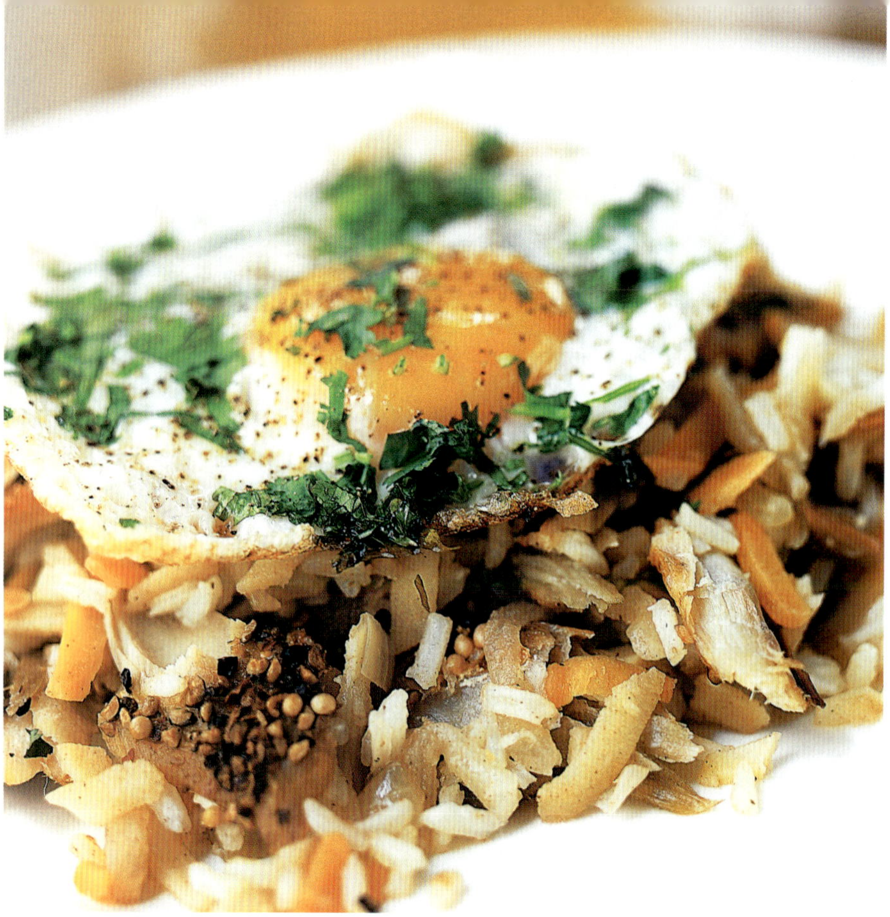

# Spiced Root Veg with Mackerel and Fried Eggs

**PER SERVING**
**547 kcalories**
**protein 22g**
**carbohydrate 65g**
**fat 24g**
**saturated fat 5g**
**fibre 5g**
**added sugar none**
**salt 1.32g**

**This delicious kedgeree-like concoction offers almost the whole 'five a day' in one dish, as well as the valuable protective qualities of the fish oils in the mackerel (see page 76).**

**PREPARATION** 5 minutes
**COOKING** 25 minutes

225g/8oz long-grain rice
2 tsp grapeseed oil
1 onion, chopped
2 large carrots, grated
4 small turnips, grated
2 large parsnips, grated
2 heaped tsp garam masala
150ml/¼ pint vegetable stock
4 small eggs
generous handful of fresh coriander leaves
2 small peppered mackerel fillets, skinned and broken into large chunks

**for the fresh mango jam**
2 tbsp good-quality mango chutney
1 small banana, peeled and cut into chunks
juice of ½ lime
1 small ripe mango, peeled, removed from the stone and cut into chunks

1 Cook the rice according to the packet instructions. Meanwhile, heat the oil in a large non-stick wok. Add the onion and cook for 5 minutes, stirring occasionally, until softened and just beginning to brown. Stir in the grated vegetables and cook, stirring, for 1 minute. Add 2 tablespoons of water and cover with a tight-fitting lid. Reduce the heat and cook for 5 minutes until softened.
2 Remove the lid, stir in the garam masala and cook for 1 minute. Stir in the stock with the cooked rice and gently heat through.
3 Meanwhile, heat a large non-stick frying pan and wipe with a little oil. Crack in the eggs, scatter over the coriander and season with black pepper. Cover with a tight-fitting lid and cook for about 2 minutes until the eggs are just set.
4 Meanwhile, make the fresh mango jam by gently folding all the ingredients together.
5 To serve, stir the mackerel into the spiced vegetables and rice, and divide between 4 serving dishes. Top each with a coriander egg and serve with mango jam.

# Ratatouille Omelette

**PER SERVING**
**252 kcalories**
**protein 12g**
**carbohydrate 7g**
**fat 20g**
**saturated fat 4g**
**fibre 3g**
**added sugar none**
**salt 0.53g**

PREPARATION about 10 minutes
COOKING 20–25 minutes

- 4 tbsp olive oil
- 1 onion, sliced
- 1 garlic clove, finely chopped
- 1 aubergine, cut into chunks
- 2 courgettes, cut into chunks
- 2 tomatoes, cut into wedges
- 6 eggs
- ½ tsp dried oregano
- handful of fresh basil leaves (optional)

1 Heat the oil in a heatproof frying pan. Add the onion and cook until softened. Add the garlic, aubergine and courgettes, and cook for about 5–8 minutes until softened and slightly brown. Add the tomato wedges and season with salt and pepper.
2 Meanwhile, preheat the grill. Beat the eggs in a bowl, stir in the dried oregano and season.
3 Pour the beaten eggs over the vegetables and cook for about 5–8 minutes, until the bottom is starting to brown and the egg looks softly set.
4 Slide the omelette under the grill until the top looks puffed and golden.
5 Tear over the basil leaves, if using, then cut the omelette into wedges and serve with a green salad.

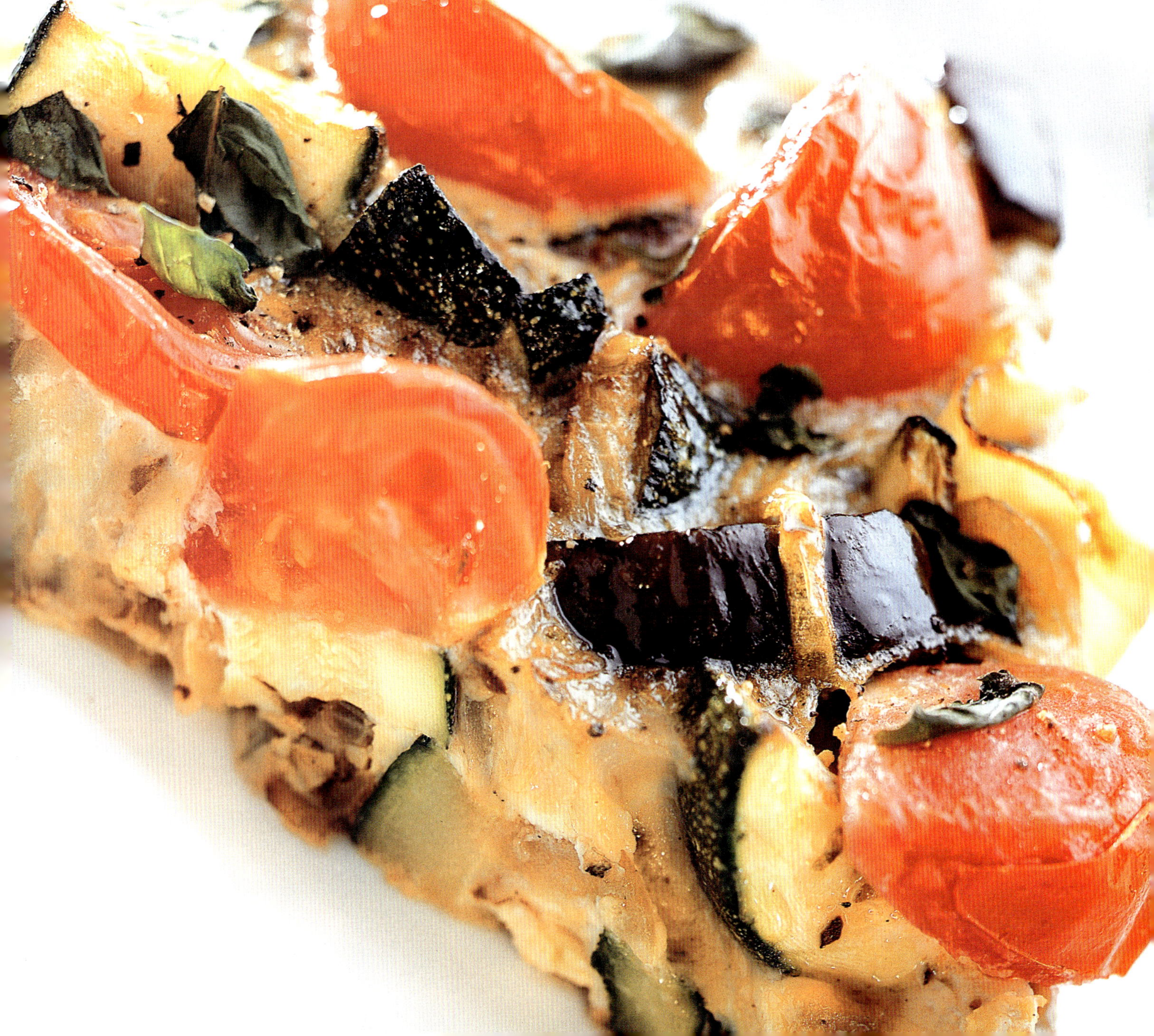

# Smoked Haddock and Leek Risotto

**Leeks are very healthy, having all the protective powers of the garlic family and the nutrients of greens.**

SERVES 6
PREPARATION 20 minutes
COOKING 25 minutes

- 900g/2lb smoked haddock
- 1.7 litres/3 pints vegetable or fish stock
- 3 large leeks, very thinly sliced
- 2 tbsp olive oil
- 25g/¾oz butter
- 500g/1lb 2oz risotto rice
- 200ml/7fl oz dry white wine
- pinch of saffron strands
- handful each chopped parsley and chives
- 30g/1oz Parmesan, freshly grated

1 Put the haddock, skin-side down, in a shallow pan. Pour over 600ml/1 pint of stock. Bring to the boil. Cover and simmer for 5 minutes until the fish is just cooked. Transfer to a plate to cool.

2 Pour the cooking liquid into a large pan with the rest of the stock and bring to the boil. Add the leeks and cook for 1–2 minutes to soften. Remove and set aside in a bowl. Keep the stock at a simmer.

3 Heat the oil and half the butter in a deep pan. Cook the rice for 5 minutes, stirring, until translucent. Increase heat, add the wine and simmer gently. When most of the wine has been absorbed, stir in all but 300ml/½ pint of the stock.

4 Cook over a moderate heat, stirring every few minutes. Add the saffron after 8 minutes. After 15 minutes, taste a grain; it should be creamy with some bite. Add some of the reserved stock if the mixture becomes too dry.

5 Skin the fish and flake into chunks. Fold the leeks, fish and any juices into the rice with the herbs, Parmesan, remaining butter and seasoning to taste.

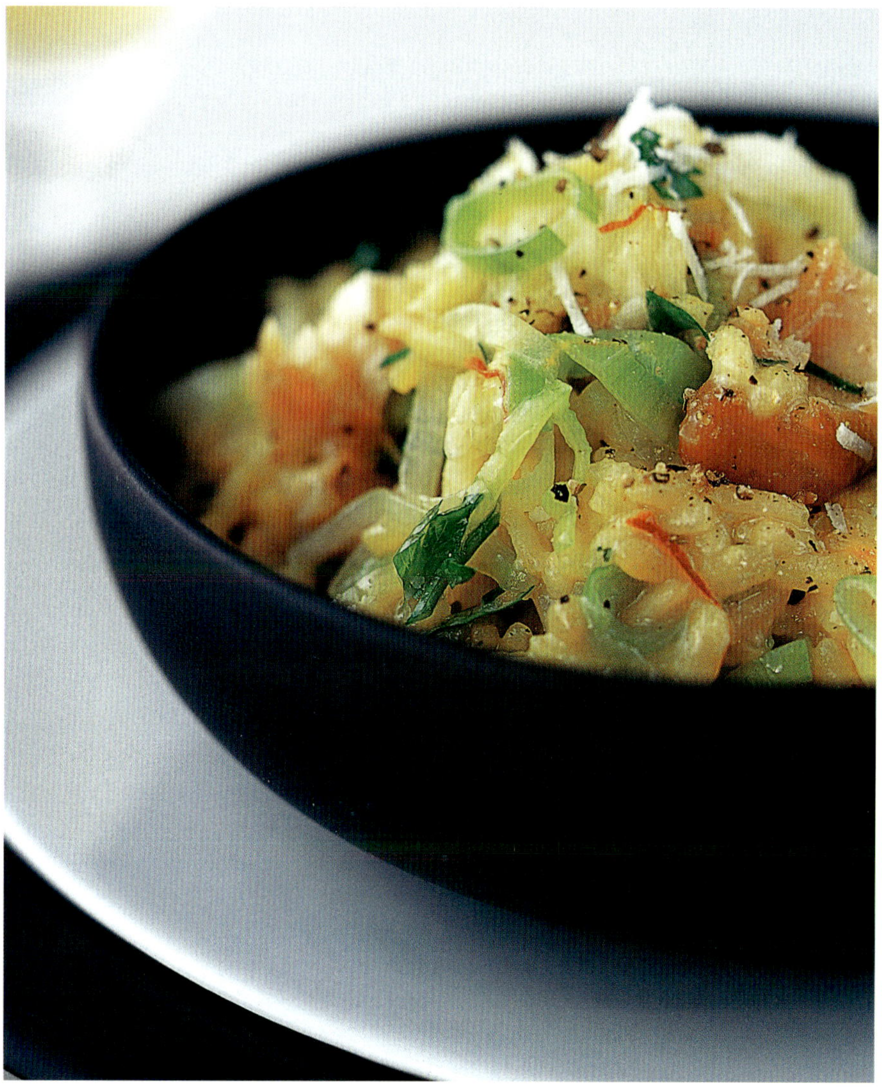

PER SERVING
**521 kcalories**
**protein 39g**
**carbohydrate 67g**
**fat 10g**
**saturated fat 4g**
**fibre 3g**
**added sugar none**
**salt 4.04g**

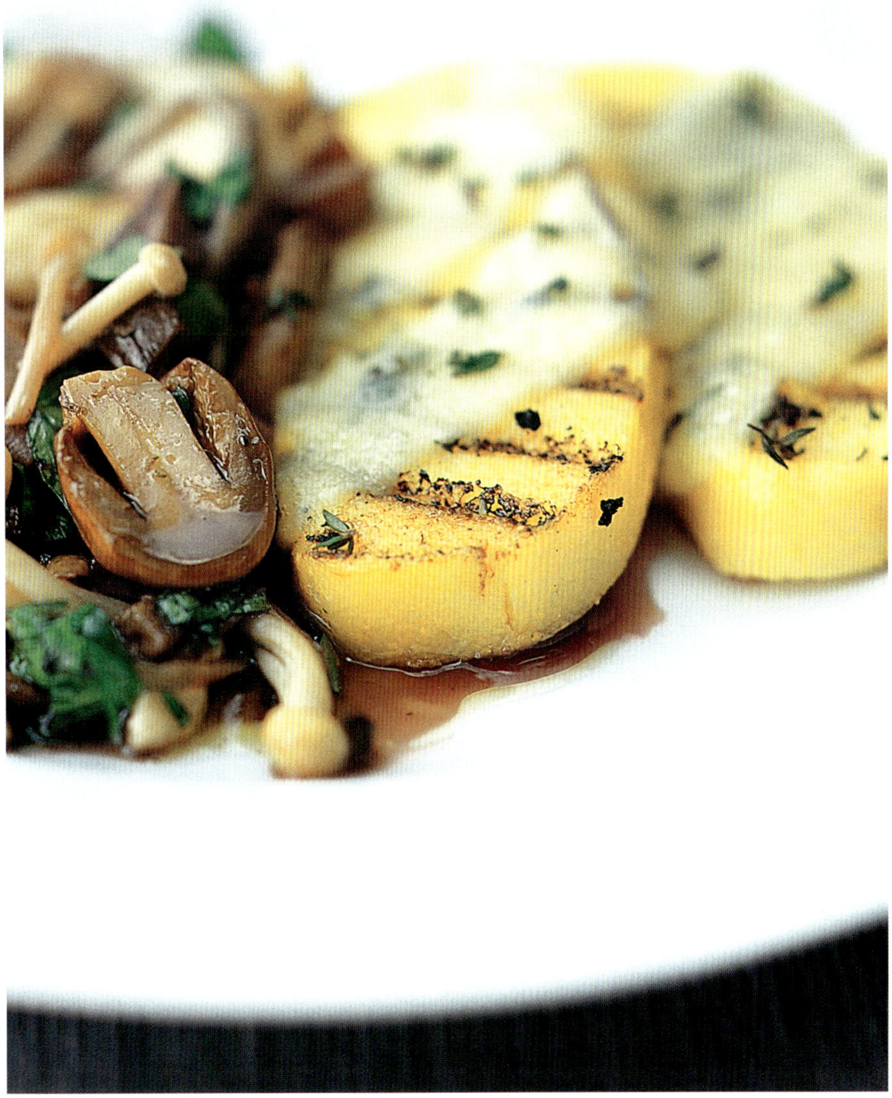

PER SERVING
346 kcalories
protein 7g
carbohydrate 22g
fat 24g
saturated fat 8g
fibre 3g
added sugar none
salt 0.93g

# Griddled Polenta with Porcini

PREPARATION 30 minutes
COOKING 35 minutes

- 15g/½oz dried ceps (porcini)
- 175ml/6fl oz warm water
- 5 tbsp olive oil
- 3 large garlic cloves, finely chopped
- 8 ready-to-use polenta slices, chilled (available from supermarket chiller cabinets, usually next to fresh pasta)
- 25g/¾oz butter
- 1 small onion, sliced
- 5-6 sprigs of fresh thyme
- 350g/12oz mushrooms, such as chestnut, shiitake and blewit, sliced
- 125ml/4fl oz red wine
- 60g/2oz Gruyère cheese, cut into thin slivers
- large handful of chopped parsley

1 Soak the ceps in the warm water for 20 minutes. Mix 3 tablespoons of the oil with one-third of the garlic. Spread this over both sides of the polenta and season. Preheat a barbecue or griddle.

2 Tip the soaked ceps into a sieve over a bowl, reserving the soaking liquid. Rinse the ceps under cold water, then chop them.

3 Melt the butter with the remaining oil in a deep frying pan, then fry the onion over a moderate heat until golden. Stir in the ceps, half the thyme and the remaining garlic. Stir-fry for another minute.

4 Add the fresh mushrooms and fry until starting to brown, then pour in the cep soaking liquid and the wine. Season well. Bring to the boil and cook over a high heat for about 2 minutes to reduce the juices. Remove from the heat and keep warm.

5 Put the polenta on the barbecue or griddle for 10 minutes until charred and crisp underneath. Turn and cook for 5 minutes, then sprinkle with the remaining thyme and top with the cheese. Cook for 5 minutes until the cheese melts.

6 Put 2 polenta slices on each plate. Stir most of the parsley into the mushrooms, then spoon them and their juices alongside the polenta. Scatter over the remaining parsley.

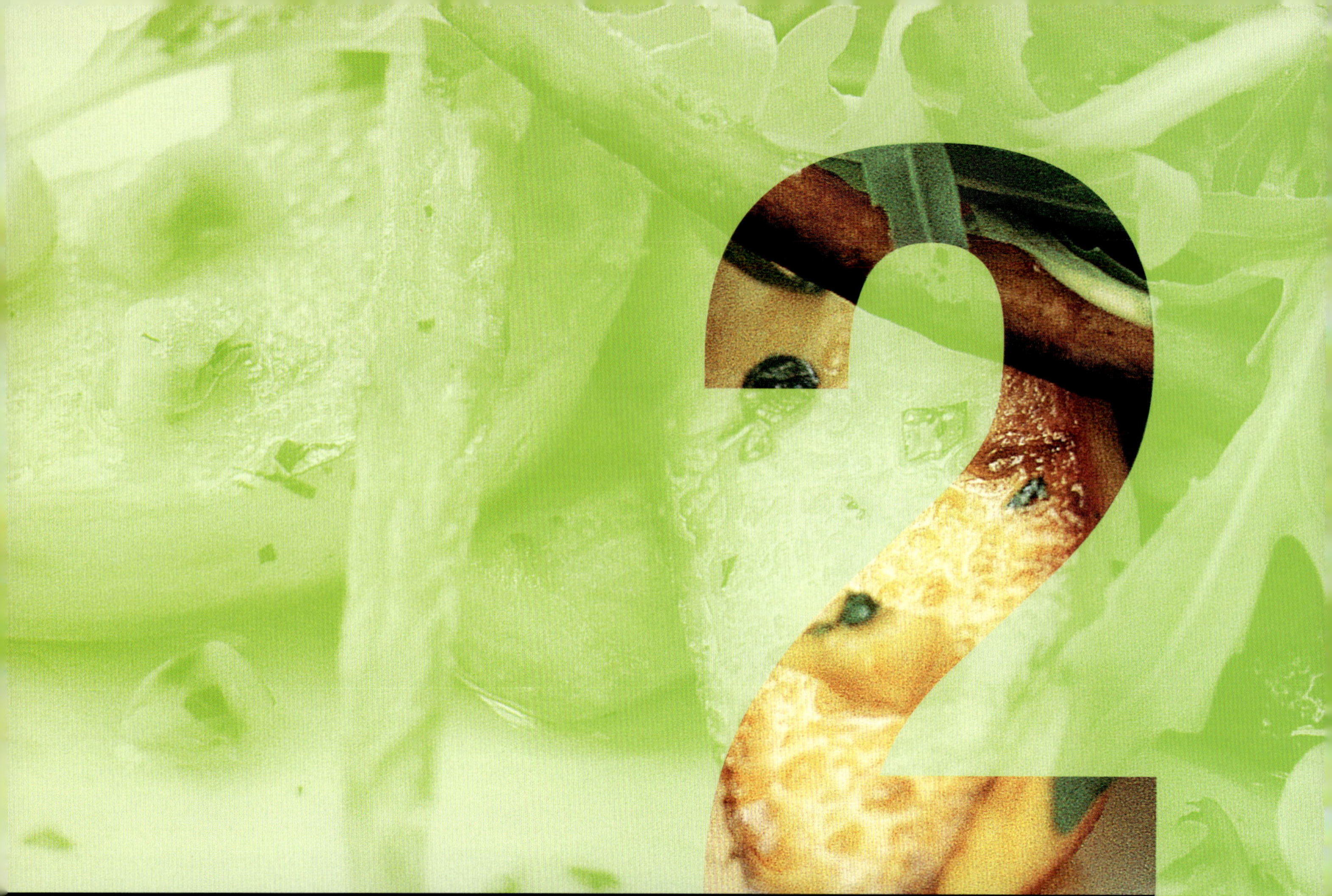

# Sound Starters and Light Meals

*In any healthy regime, rather than eliminating starters in an effort to reduce your calorie intake, they can quite readily form a useful means of boosting your vegetable and fruit intake to take you towards your 'five a day'. They are also a very good way of ensuring that you get your daily measure of many beneficial foods, like oily fish or pulses. Always try to ensure that your snacks and light meals are as balanced as they possibly can be, with just a little protein and lots of complex carbohydrates.*

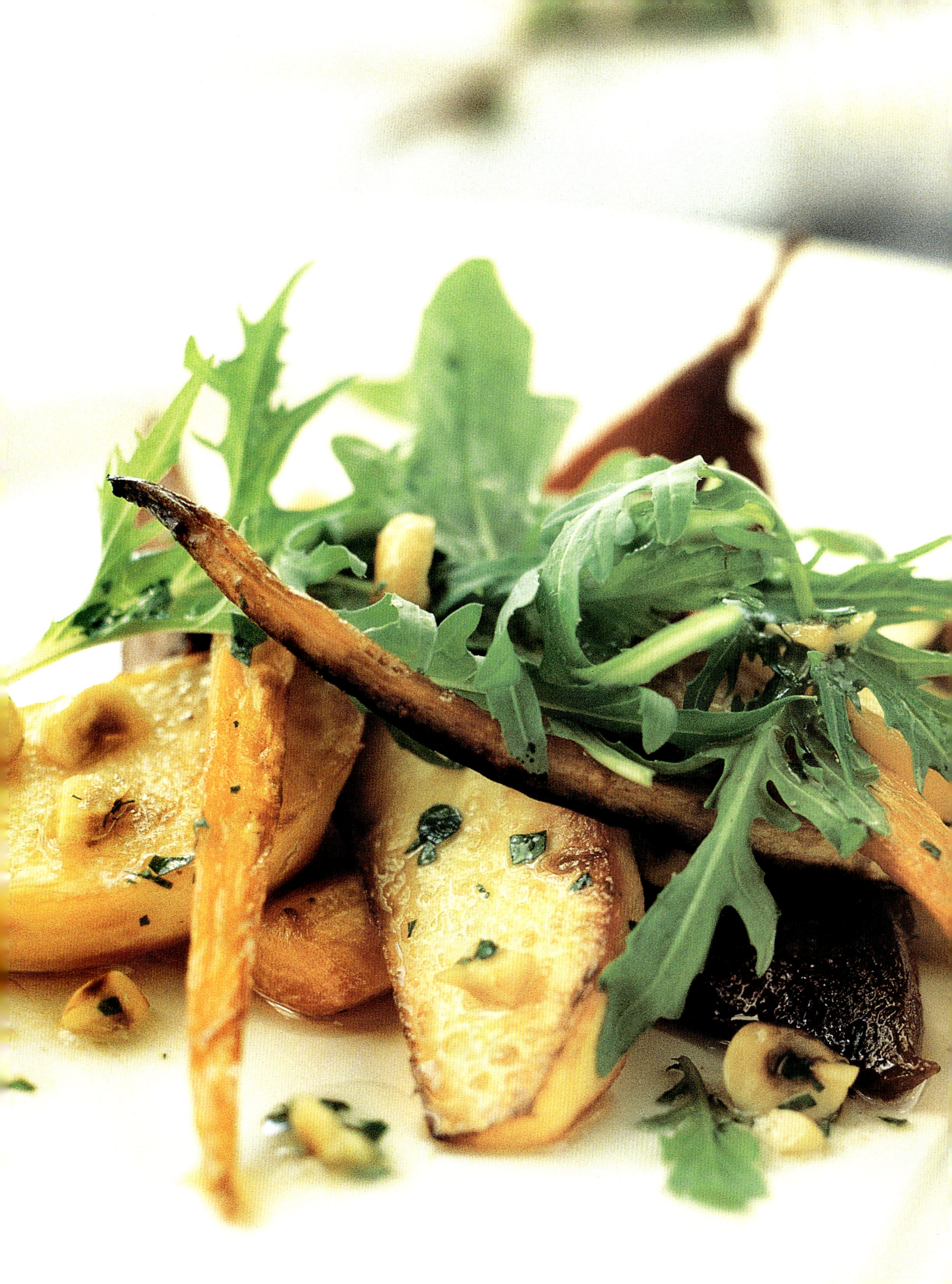

# Salad of Braised Winter Vegetables with Toasted Hazelnut Dressing

**It's best to serve the finished vegetables at room temperature, or even just take the chill off them in the microwave.**

SERVES 6
PREPARATION 25 minutes
COOKING 40 minutes, plus 1 hour for the beetroot

1 medium uncooked beetroot
1 small swede
2 small turnips
½ small celeriac
2 carrots
2 medium parsnips
about 150ml/¼ pint extra-virgin olive oil, for braising, plus 1 tbsp for frying
juice of ½ lemon
100g/4oz salad leaves (be adventurous and try using lamb's lettuce, escarole or batavia)

**for the dressing**
60g/2oz hazelnuts
2 tsp Dijon mustard
2 tsp sherry vinegar
3 tbsp vegetable oil
4 tsp hazelnut oil
1 tbsp chopped fresh flat-leaf parsley

PER SERVING
**441 kcalories • protein 4g • carbohydrate 18g fat 40g • saturated fat 5g • fibre 8g added sugar none • salt 0.51g**

1 Wash the beetroot well and cut the stalk down by about 2cm/¾inch. Don't cut off the root as it stops the beetroot 'bleeding' while it's cooking. Put the beetroot in a pan, cover with cold water, add a pinch of salt and bring to the boil. Reduce the heat and simmer for about 1 hour until tender – you should be able to push a small sharp knife straight through the centre easily. Allow to cool in the water, then peel and cut into wedges.
2 Preheat the oven to 200°C/400°F/Gas 6. Peel all the remaining vegetables and cut them so that they keep a certain amount of their natural shape – cut the swede, turnips and celeriac into wedges and the carrots and parsnips into long shards, but don't slice them too thinly or they will burn during braising.
3 Tip all the vegetables into a deep flameproof and ovenproof dish or casserole and pour over just enough oil barely to cover them. Season well with salt and pepper, add a squeeze of lemon juice and heat on the hob until the oil is hot (don't overheat the oil, though – remember this is braising not deep-frying). Cover tightly with a lid or foil and cook in the oven for 20–30 minutes, until the vegetables are tender but not overcooked. Using a slotted spoon, remove the vegetables from the oil and drain well. Allow to cool. (Use the leftover oil for salad dressings or reuse for cooking – you could even use it to braise more vegetables.)
4 Make the dressing: preheat the grill, put the hazelnuts on a baking sheet and grill for 3–4 minutes until the skins are dry and shrivelled. Put the nuts in a clean tea towel and rub to remove the skins. When the nuts are cool enough to handle, chop them roughly.
5 Put the mustard in a bowl and add the vinegar. Gradually whisk in the vegetable oil so the dressing emulsifies and thickens, then add the hazelnut oil and parsley. Season and stir in the chopped hazelnuts.
6 Just before serving, heat a tablespoon of olive oil in a large frying pan, add the vegetables and cook for about 5 minutes, stirring occasionally until they are lightly browned. (You may have to do this in batches.) Remove them from the pan and keep at room temperature.
7 Season the salad leaves with salt and pepper, and add enough of the dressing to coat the leaves. Arrange the braised vegetables on serving plates, drizzle over a little more of the hazelnut dressing and pile the dressed leaves on top.

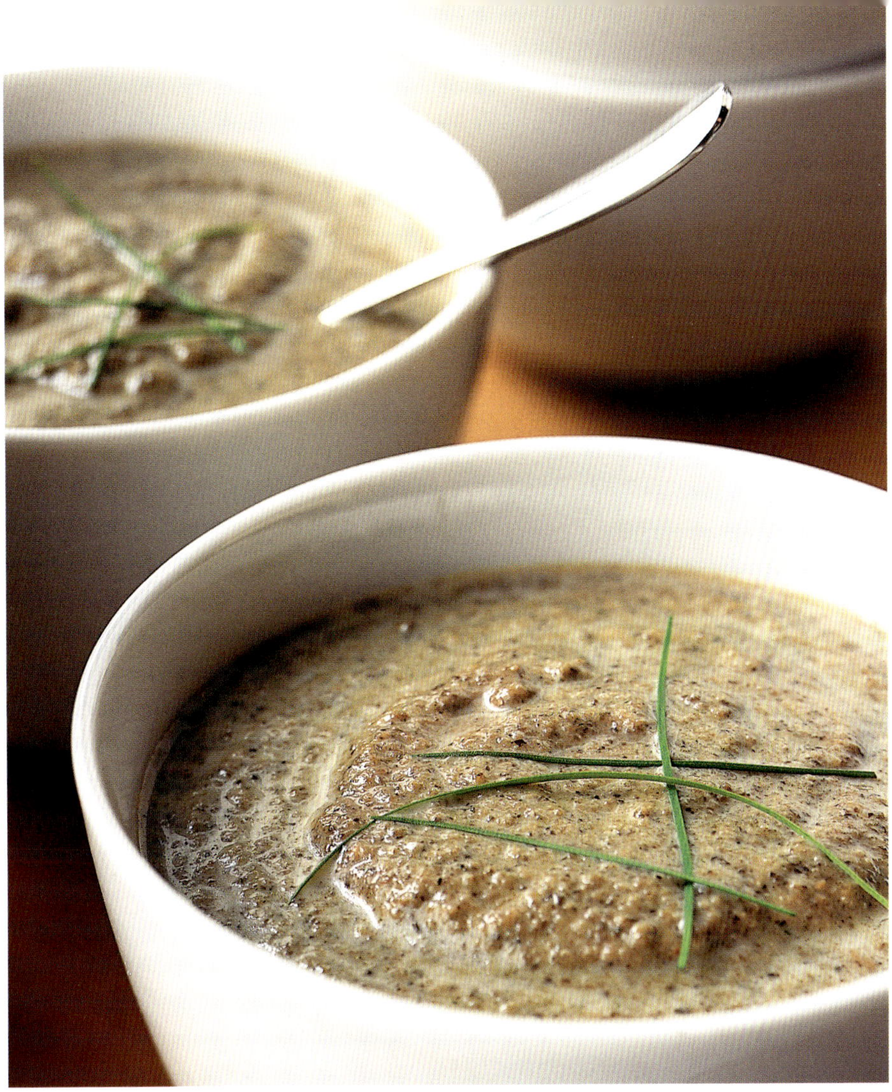

PER SERVING
169 kcalories
protein 3g
carbohydrate 3g
fat 15g
saturated fat 9g
fibre 1g
added sugar none
salt 0.90g

# Cream of Mushroom Soup

**Home-made cream of mushroom soup is a real treat. A few dried porcini add a rich autumnal note, and a splash of white wine brings the flavours together quite magically. The soup's creamy texture comes from the liquidized fungi, so it really does need only a spot of cream. It is often forgotten that mushrooms are nutritious, containing a variety of B vitamins, as well as potassium and copper.**

SERVES 6
PREPARATION 10 minutes
COOKING 30 minutes

60g/2oz butter
2 garlic cloves, chopped
4 tbsp finely chopped fresh parsley
450g/1lb chestnut or white mushrooms (caps or flats, not buttons), roughly chopped
15g/½oz dried porcini
150ml/¼ pint dry white wine
juice of ½ lemon
1 litre/1¾ pints chicken or vegetable stock
6 tbsp double cream

1 Melt the butter in a large pan, then add the garlic, parsley, chopped mushrooms and dried porcini. Cook over a moderate heat, stirring, until the mushrooms have reabsorbed the liquid they release. Be careful not to let the garlic or mushrooms brown. Add the wine and cook over a high heat until it has almost disappeared, then add the lemon juice and stock. Bring to the boil, reduce to a simmer and season with salt and pepper. Simmer uncovered for 20 minutes.
2 Liquidize the soup in a food processor or blender. Rinse the pan and pour the soup back in. Stir in the cream and season again if necessary.
3 To serve, reheat gently, being careful not to allow the soup to boil.

# Aubergine and Mozzarella Stacks

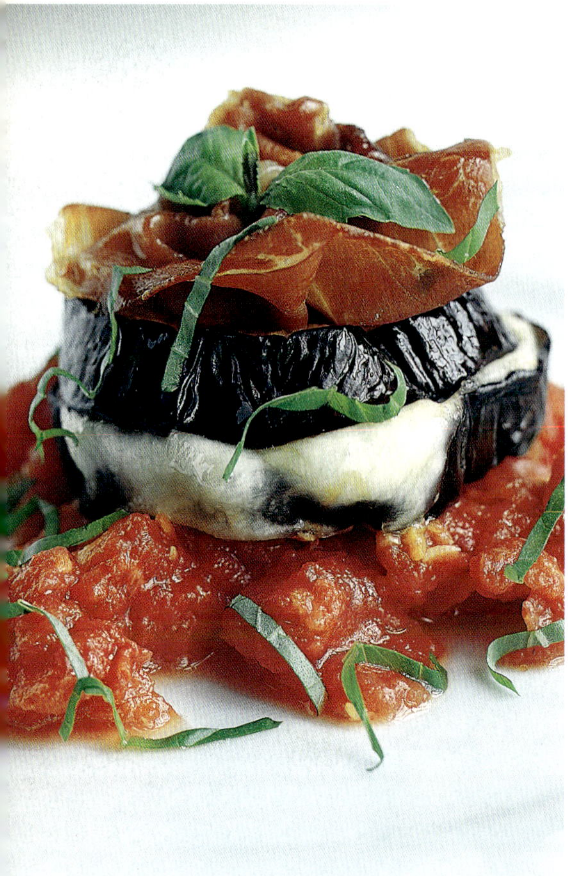

**Crushed tomatoes, or passata, are available in jars in larger supermarkets. If you can't get them, use good-quality canned chopped tomatoes, as cheaper ones tend to be watery. Mozzarella is fairly low in fat for a cheese, about 30% less than most hard cheeses and half that of cream cheese. Serve the stacks with garlic bread.**

SERVES 6
PREPARATION 20 minutes
COOKING 20–25 minutes

1 medium aubergine
2 tbsp olive oil, plus more for the dish
150g/5oz pack of mozzarella
6 slices of prosciutto
handful of basil leaves, torn, to serve

**for the sauce**

350g/12oz jar of crushed tomatoes, or
400g/14oz can of chopped tomatoes and 2 tsp tomato purée
2 tbsp extra-virgin olive oil
1 garlic clove, chopped

PER SERVING
**192 kcalories • protein 13g • carbohydrate 3g fat 15g • saturated fat 5g •fibre 1g added sugar none • salt 1.25g**

1 Preheat the oven to 200°C/400°F/Gas 6. Cut twelve 1cm/½in aubergine slices and put them over the grill pan in one layer. Brush with half the olive oil and grill for 3–4 minutes. Turn over, brush and grill again, then leave to cool.

2 Cut the mozzarella into 6 slices. Sandwich each between 2 aubergine slices and put in a greased shallow ovenproof dish. Crumple a slice of prosciutto on top of each 'sandwich'. Bake for 12–15 minutes until the cheese melts.

3 Meanwhile, make the sauce: put all the ingredients in a pan and simmer briefly (or until slightly thickened, if using canned tomatoes). Spoon a little sauce on each plate, put the stacks on top and scatter with basil.

# Leafy Artichoke and Crisp Prosciutto Salad

PER SERVING
**221 kcalories
protein 9g
carbohydrate 2g
fat 20g
saturated fat 4g
fibre trace
added sugar 1g
salt 1.5g**

SERVES 6
PREPARATION 15 minutes

**As well as their being a good source of folate and potassium, artichokes contain a compound called cynarin that is said to improve liver function.**

275g/10oz jar of artichokes in oil
a little olive oil
12 slices of prosciutto, each cut into three pieces
large bag of small-leaf salad (about 150–200g/5–7oz)
crusty bread, to serve

**for the dressing**

1 tsp clear honey
1 tsp Dijon or wholegrain mustard
2 tbsp wine vinegar
6 tbsp olive oil

1 Tip the artichokes into a sieve to drain, then slice them. Heat a little olive oil in a large frying pan, then fry the prosciutto pieces quickly in batches over a high heat until crisp. Drain on kitchen paper. Tip the salad leaves into a large bowl.

2 Make the dressing: put the honey, mustard, vinegar, salt and pepper in a bowl and whisk well until thickened. Gradually whisk in the olive oil. Taste and season if necessary.

3 Just before serving, add the artichoke slices to the leaves and toss in the dressing. Divide between 6 side plates and pile the crisp prosciutto on top. Serve with warm crusty bread.

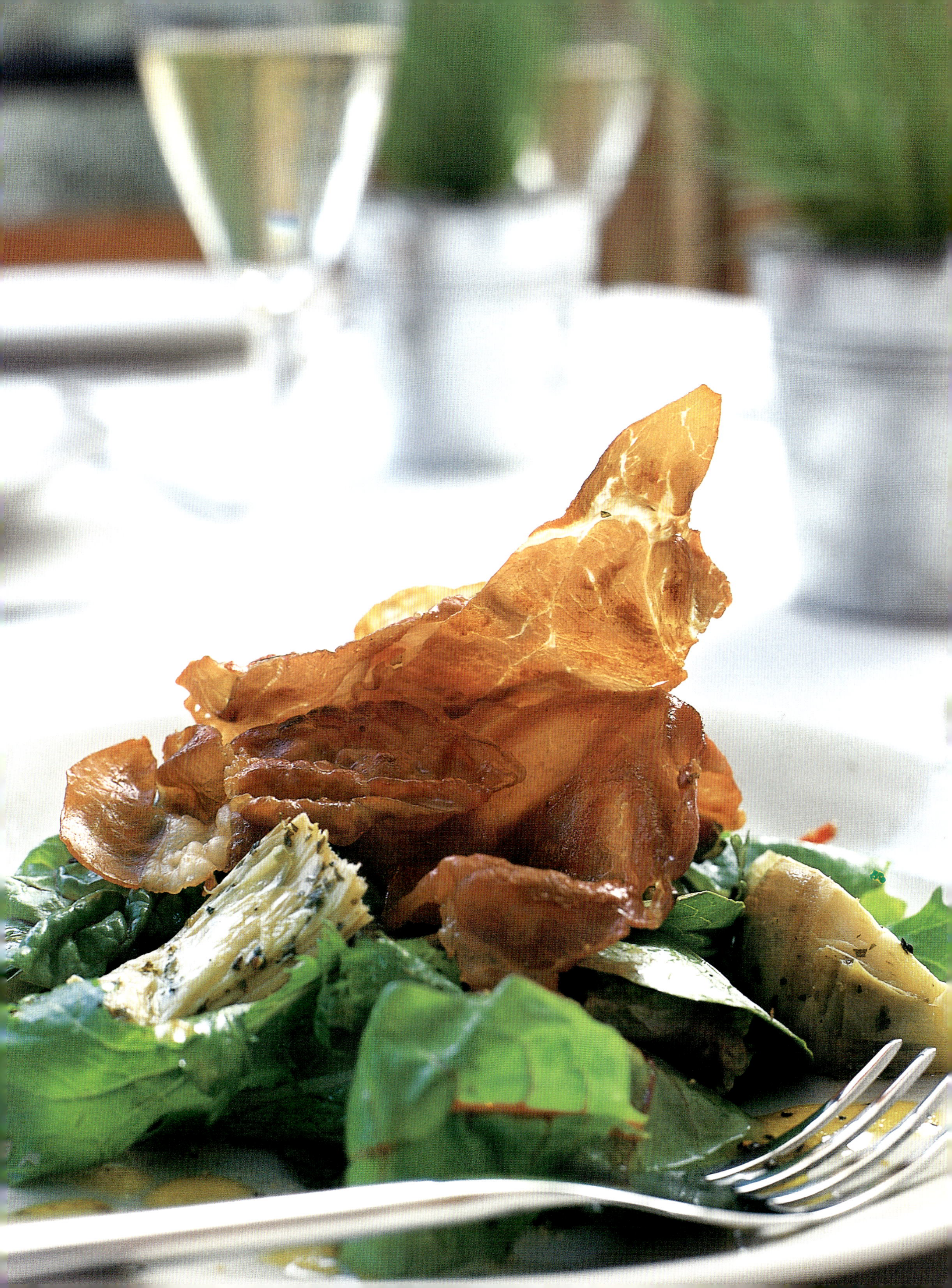

# Balsamic Onion and Goats' Cheese Salad

PER SERVING
112 kcalories
protein 5g
carbohydrate 11g
fat 6g
saturated fat trace
fibre 2g
added sugar 2g
salt 0.32g

**Onions are often overlooked, both in terms of their flavour and as health-givers. As much a 'superfood' as their close relative garlic, they have all the same powers of blood-thinning and cholesterol reduction, as well as helping to relieve the symptoms of colds and 'flus. The onions can be cooked the day before, then put into an oven pre-heated to 200°C/400°F/Gas 6 for 15 minutes just before serving.**

PREPARATION 5 minutes
COOKING about 40 minutes

3 onions
2 tsp olive oil
2 thyme sprigs
4 garlic cloves
1 tsp light muscovado sugar
3 tbsp balsamic vinegar
4 handfuls of mixed salad leaves
100g/4oz soft goats' cheese

1 Quarter the onions lengthwise, keeping the roots intact on each quarter.
2 Heat the olive oil in a frying pan and add the onions to the pan, along with the thyme sprigs and garlic cloves. Cover with a lid and cook for 12–15 minutes, stirring occasionally, until the onions are softened and beginning to brown.
3 Sprinkle over the muscovado sugar, cover again and cook for a further 10 minutes, stirring, until the onions are beginning to caramelize. (Keep an eye on the heat – if it gets too hot, add a splash of water to prevent the onions from burning.)
4 Add the balsamic vinegar. Stir, season, cover and cook for 15 minutes until most of the vinegar has bubbled away and the onions are sticky. Remove the lid, add 3 table-spoons of water and stir to lift the pan juices. The onions should be very tender.
5 Pile a handful of mixed salad leaves on to each of 4 plates and arrange the onions on top. Crumble over the goats' cheese and drizzle with the pan juices. Serve warm.

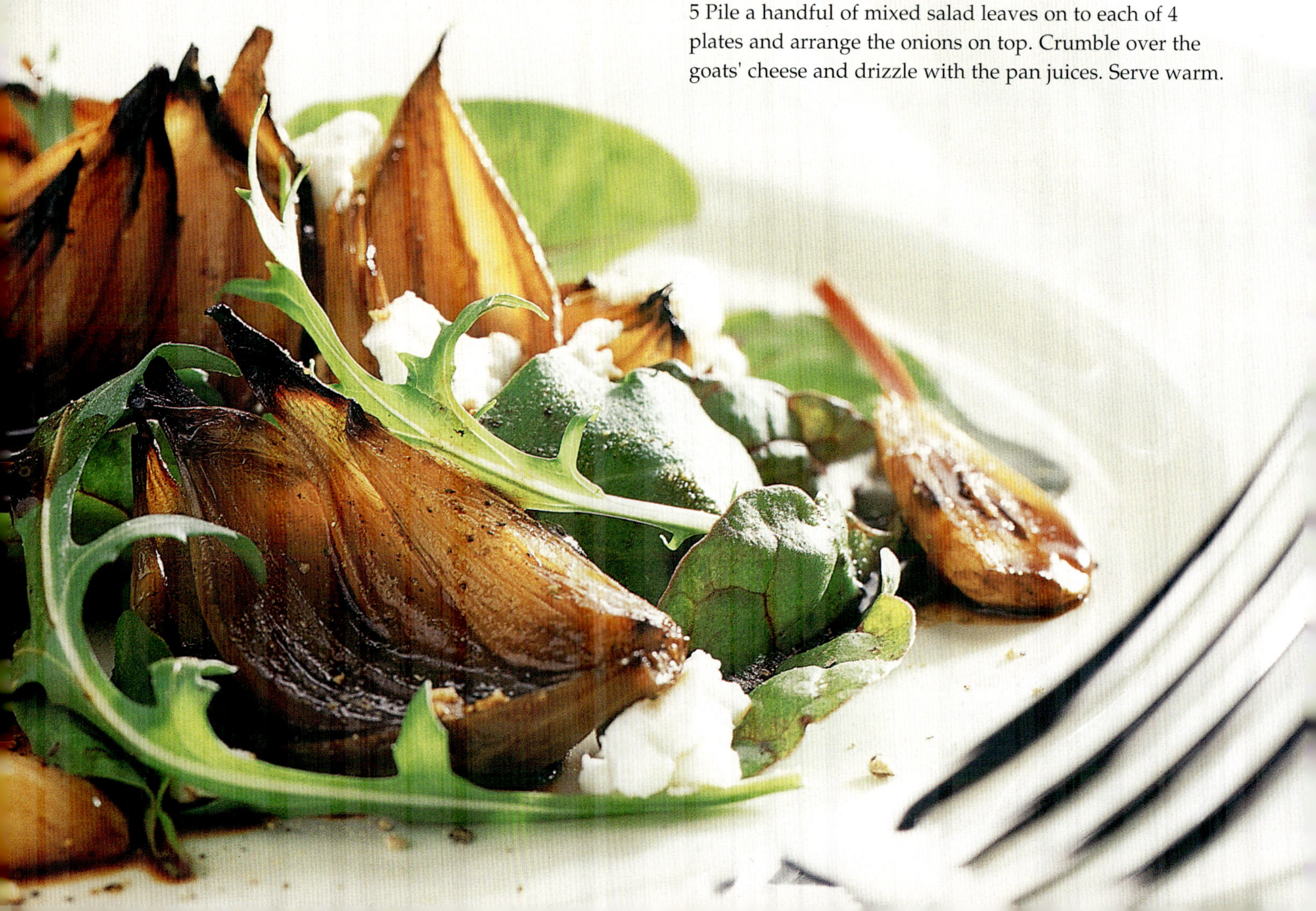

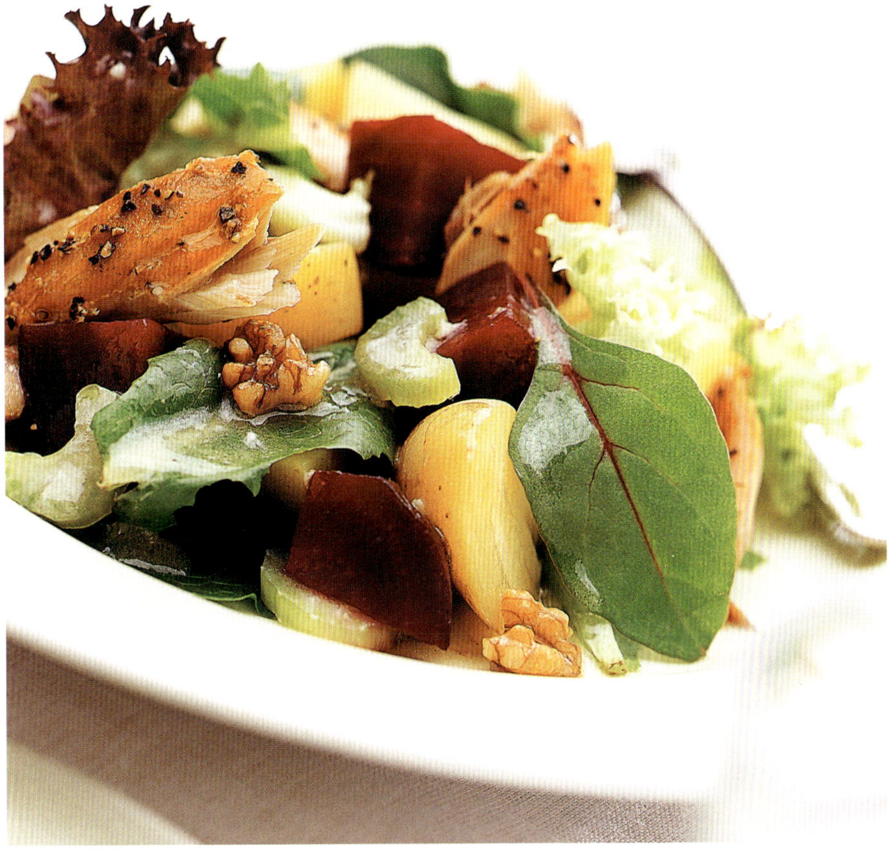

PER SERVING
634 kcalories
protein 22g
carbohydrate 26g
fat 50g
saturated fat 2g
fibre 4g
added sugar none
salt 1.91g

# Warm Mackerel and Beetroot Salad

**Although this tasty and colourful salad is quite high in fat, it is mostly unsaturated – and a large part of it in the form of healthy fish oils. Otherwise, with these protective fish oils, the raw goodness of the mixed salad leaves, the rich vitamin and mineral content of the beetroot and walnuts, and the blood-pressure-reducing phytochemicals of the celery, it couldn't be much healthier.**

PREPARATION about 10 minutes
COOKING 12–15 minutes

450g/1lb new potatoes, cut into bite-sized pieces
3 smoked mackerel fillets, skinned
250g/9oz cooked beetroot
120g/4oz bag of mixed salad leaves
2 celery stalks, thinly sliced
60g/2oz walnut pieces

**for the dressing**

3 tbsp walnut oil
2 tbsp sunflower oil
2 tbsp fresh lemon juice
2 tsp creamed horseradish sauce

1 Cook the potatoes in boiling salted water for 12–15 minutes until just tender. Drain and set aside. Flake the mackerel fillets into large pieces. Cut the beetroot into bite-sized pieces.

2 Make the dressing by mixing together all the ingredients; season.

3 Tip the salad leaves into a bowl. Add the potatoes, mackerel, beetroot, celery and walnuts. Pour over the dressing and toss well. Serve warm.

# Watermelon, Prawn and Cucumber Salad

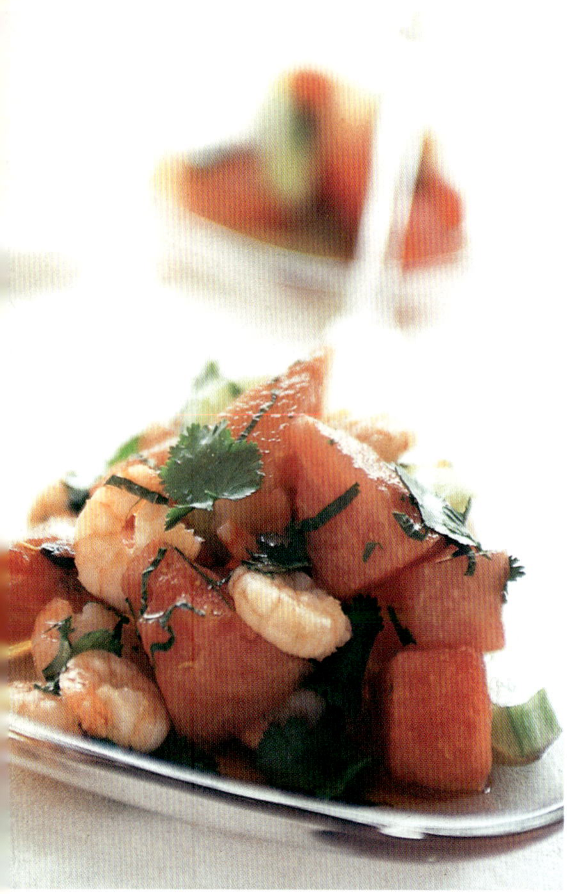

**This colourful salad makes a wonderfully refreshing summer starter, containing virtually no fat at all.**

SERVES 6
PREPARATION 30 minutes

1.35kg/3lb watermelon, seeds removed (about ½ a small one)
1 large cucumber, peeled
225g/8oz peeled cooked tiger prawns
small handful of fresh mint leaves, roughly chopped
small handful of fresh coriander leaves, roughly chopped

**for the dressing**

2 tbsp palm sugar or light muscovado sugar
juice of 1 lime
1 tbsp white rum
¼ tsp Angostura bitters

PER SERVING
**114 kcalories • protein 9g • carbohydrate 17g • fat 1g • saturated fat none • fibre 1g • added sugar 7g • salt 0.51g**

1 First make the dressing: put the sugar in a small bowl, add the lime juice and stir until the sugar has dissolved, then add the rum and Angostura bitters.
2 Cut the watermelon into 4 wedges and remove the rind. Cut the flesh into 2.5cm/1in chunks and pat dry with kitchen paper. Transfer to a large bowl.
3 Halve the cucumber lengthwise and scoop out the seeds. Cut the flesh at an angle into 1cm/½in slices and add to the melon together with the prawns.
4 Just before serving, pour over the dressing and most of the herbs. Toss well and divide between 6 plates and scatter over the remaining herbs to serve.

# Smoked Trout and Dill Blinis

PER SERVING
**165 kcalories**
**protein 10g**
**carbohydrate 11g**
**fat 9g**
**saturated fat 5g**
**fibre trace**
**added sugar 1g**
**salt 0.3g**

**Blinis are sold in the chill cabinet of many supermarkets.**

SERVES 6
PREPARATION 5 minutes
COOKING 6–8 minutes

225g/8oz smoked trout fillets (usually vacuum-packed)
100ml/3½fl oz crème fraîche
1 tbsp chopped fresh dill, plus more, roughly chopped, to garnish
2 tsp fresh lemon juice
6 ready-made large blinis or 18 small ones
small jar of black herring roe

1 Break the smoked trout into bite-sized pieces (the easiest way to do this is with your hands). In a small bowl, mix together the crème fraîche, chopped dill and lemon juice, then season with salt and pepper.
2 Just before serving, toast the blinis on each side. Put one on each plate (or 3 if you're using small ones) and top with a spoonful of the mixture, then some trout pieces, followed by a spoonful of the herring roe. Garnish with roughly chopped dill and serve immediately.

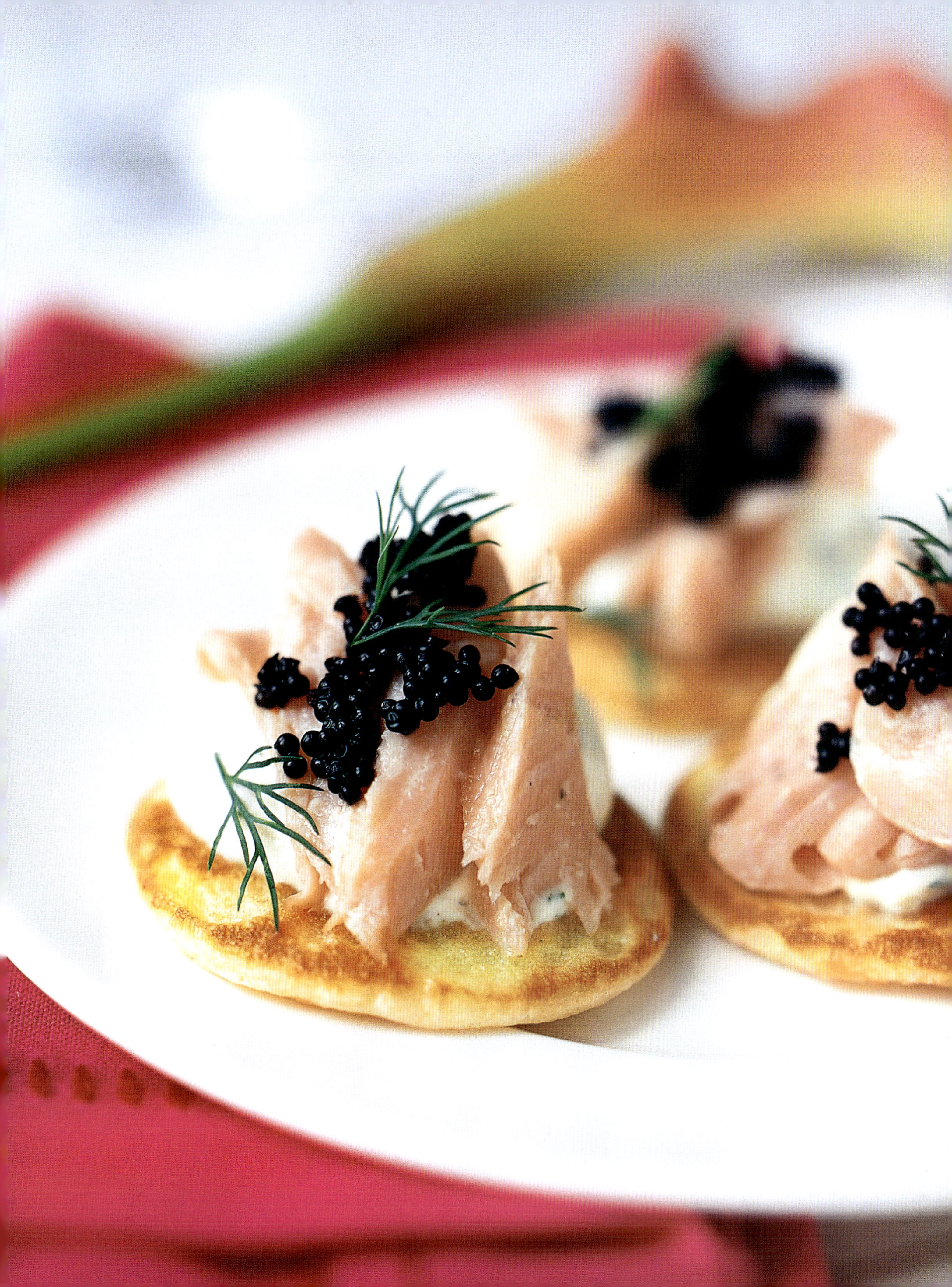

# Spice'n'sizzle Prawns on Black-eyed Bean Salsa

20 raw king prawns in the shell, heads removed
½ tsp mild chilli powder
pinch of ground cinnamon
1 tbsp olive oil, plus more to serve
coriander sprigs and chilli powder, to garnish
lime wedges, to serve

**for the Black-eyed Bean Salsa**

1 small red onion, finely chopped
1 red chilli, finely chopped (deseeded if you want it mild, with the seeds if you like it hot)
1 garlic clove, finely chopped
400g/14oz can of black-eyed beans, drained
handful of fresh coriander, roughly chopped
1 tbsp clear honey
grated zest and juice of 1 lime
grated zest and juice of 1 small lemon

**From the moment this hits your mouth, your taste buds are in for a treat – a sensational explosion of hot chillies, cut with a touch of honey sweetness, a juicy lemon and lime sourness, and just a hint of spice. The raw vegetables and black-eyed beans of the salsa make this low-fat dish nutrient-rich.**

1 First make the salsa: mix all the ingredients together and season to taste. (If you prefer the salsa sweeter, add an extra spoonful or so of the honey.) Set aside in a cool place.
2 Shell the prawns, leaving the tail tips on, and pull out the dark intestinal vein along the back of each prawn. Toss the prawns with the chilli, cinnamon and olive oil.
3 Heat a dry non-stick pan and stir-fry the prawns for 2–3 minutes until they have just changed colour. Immediately remove the pan from the heat and tip the prawns into a bowl.
4 Spoon some salsa on to each of 4 serving plates and pile the prawns on top of it. Drizzle over a little more olive oil, garnish with some coriander sprigs and a light dusting of chilli, and serve with lime wedges.

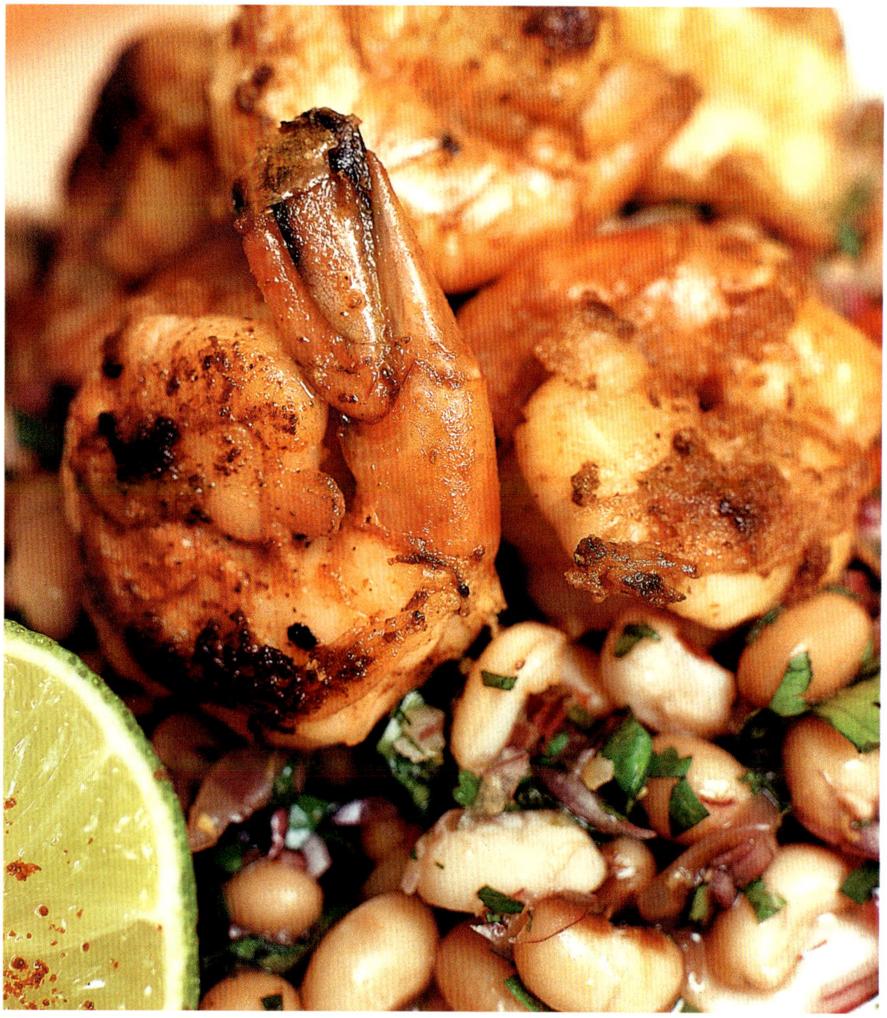

PER SERVING
**204 kcalories**
**protein 24g**
**carbohydrate 19g**
**fat 4g**
**saturated fat trace**
**fibre 2g**
**added sugar 4g**
**salt 0.74g**

PREPARATION
about 15 minutes
COOKING
2–3 minutes

# Gravadlax

900g/2lb salmon, cut into two fillets, skin left on
2 tbsp sea salt flakes
2 tbsp sugar
1 tsp coarsely crushed peppercorns (white or black, or a mixture)
1 tbsp brandy
bunch of fresh dill, coarsely chopped, plus more fresh dill sprigs to garnish
lemon wedges, to garnish
**for the mustard sauce**
2 tbsp Dijon mustard
1 tbsp sugar
2 tbsp white wine vinegar
125ml/4fl oz olive oil
2 tbsp crème fraîche or soured cream
2 tbsp chopped fresh dill

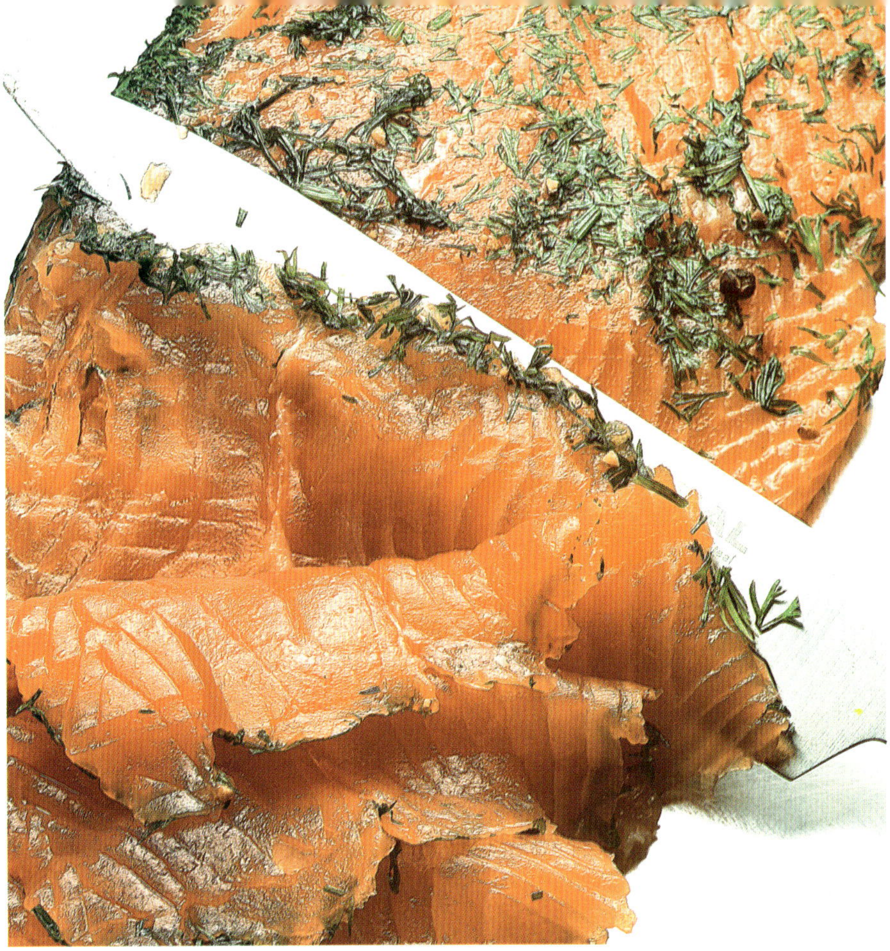

PER SERVING FOR 12:
**250 kcalories**
**protein 14g**
**carbohydrate 3g**
**fat 16g**
**saturated fat 4g**
**fibre trace**
**added sugar 3g**
**salt 7.4g**

SERVES 12 as a starter or 8 as a light main course
PREPARATION about 40 minutes, plus 2–5 days' curing

**Gravadlax, or gravlax, being only lightly cured and not smoked, retains most of the superfood qualities of fresh salmon (the beneficial omega-3 oils as well as a wide range of vitamins and minerals) with none of the possible attendant carcinogenic risk of smoking the fish. Ask for the fish to be cut into 2 fillets with the skin left on.**

1 Run your finger down the flesh of each fillet to find any stray bones. Remove any you feel, using tweezers or the point of a sharp knife.
2 Mix the salt, sugar and pepper. Use your hands to rub this mixture all over the fish. Lightly sprinkle the flesh side only with half the brandy. Sprinkle a quarter of the dill into a shallow china or glass dish large enough to take the fish comfortably. Put one salmon fillet skin-side down in the dish. Sprinkle the flesh side of both fillets with half the remaining dill and the remaining brandy. Sandwich the salmon fillets, flesh-side together, so that it looks like a whole fish again. Finish by sprinkling with the remaining dill.
3 Cover the salmon with cling film and set a large flat plate on top. Weigh this down with weights or full cans (canned beans or tomatoes – whatever comes to hand). Leave for 2–5 days in the fridge, turning the whole salmon over after day 1. The longer you leave it, the firmer the texture will be and the richer the flavour, but after 5 days it must be sliced.
4 Discard the bits of dill, which by now will be wilted, and put the salmon fillets skin-side down on a board. To serve, cut at an angle into thin slices, starting at the tail end. Work slowly and patiently (set aside a good 10 minutes for this) to try to make the slices similar in shape and size.
5 Making the mustard sauce is a doddle (and it is also a very good sauce for fresh salmon): whisk together the mustard, sugar, vinegar, salt and pepper. Continue whisking, adding the oil in a steady stream until you have a thick sauce. Fold in the crème fraîche and dill.
6 Serve the gravadlax slices (about 3 per person) on plates adorned with the sauce, and garnished with dill sprigs and the lemon wedges. Hand round black pepper.

# Oriental Prawn Tagliatelle Salad

**Fresh tagliatelle is enriched with eggs, boosting its nutritive value.**

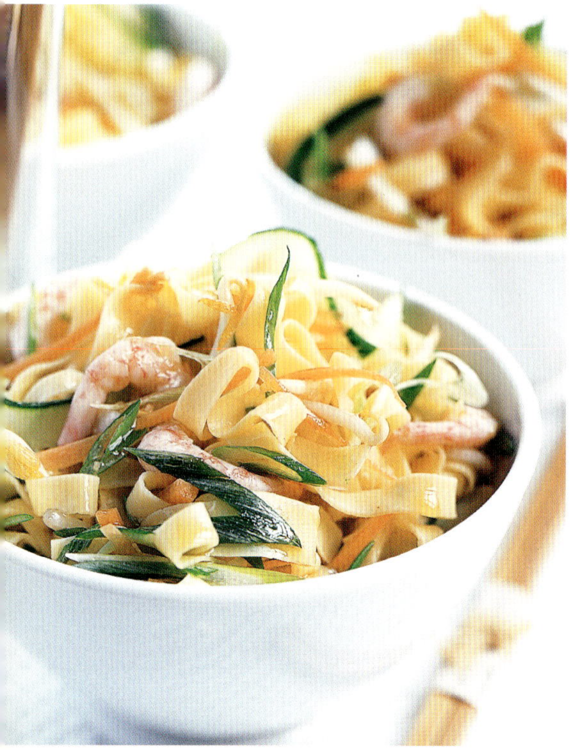

PREPARATION 20 minutes
COOKING 5–10 minutes

250g/9oz tagliatelle
100g/4oz fresh beansprouts
1 bunch of spring onions, cut into shreds
2 carrots, cut into thin sticks
¼ cucumber, cut into thin ribbons
225g/8oz cooked peeled prawns
sesame oil, for drizzling

**for the dressing**

5 tbsp sunflower oil
2 tbsp light soy sauce
2 tbsp rice vinegar or white wine vinegar
1 tbsp finely chopped fresh root ginger
1 large garlic clove, crushed
1 tsp clear honey

PER SERVING
**439 kcalories • protein 21g • carbohydrate 54g fat 17g • saturated fat 2g • fibre 4g added sugar 1g • salt 3.42g**

1 Cook the pasta in a pan of boiling salted water until tender but still firm to the bite. Meanwhile, put the beansprouts in a bowl, cover with cold water and leave for 10 minutes, then drain (this crisps them up).
2 Tip the cooked pasta into a colander and cool under cold running water, then allow to drain.
3 Toss the pasta with the beansprouts, spring onions, carrots, cucumber and prawns.
4 Make the dressing by whisking all the ingredients together.
5 Pour the dressing over the pasta and lightly toss to coat. Drizzle a little sesame oil over to serve

# Roasted Pepper and Prosciutto Spaghetti Salad

PER SERVING
**428 kcalories**
**protein 14g**
**carbohydrate 50g**
**fat 21g**
**saturated fat 3g**
**fibre 3g**
**added sugar none**
**salt 1.1g**

PREPARATION 10 minutes
COOKING 40 minutes

2 red peppers, cored, deseeded and cut in quarters
1 red onion, cut into wedges
6 tbsp olive oil
225g/8oz spaghetti
1 tbsp cider or white wine vinegar
3 garlic cloves, sliced
10–12 fresh sage leaves
85g/3oz pieces of prosciutto

1 Preheat the oven to 220°C/425°F/Gas 7. Put the peppers, skin-side up, and the onion wedges in a single layer in a roasting tin. Drizzle over a tablespoon of the oil and roast for 20–30 minutes until the peppers and onions are charred (the onions will be ready slightly earlier).
2 Seal the peppers in a plastic bag and leave for 20 minutes. Meanwhile, break the spaghetti into shorter lengths, then cook in boiling salted water until tender but still firm to the bite. Drain well.
3 Make a dressing by whisking 3 tablespoons of the oil with the vinegar, and salt and pepper to taste.
4 Heat the remaining oil in a small frying pan. Quickly fry the garlic and sage for a few seconds until the garlic is golden and the sage is crisp and slightly darkened. Remove and drain on kitchen paper. Fry the prosciutto in the hot pan for a few seconds, turning constantly, until crisp. Remove and drain on kitchen paper.
5 Peel and discard the pepper skins, then tear the flesh into thin strips. Toss the pasta with the peppers, onion, garlic, sage, prosciutto and dressing. Season and serve warm.

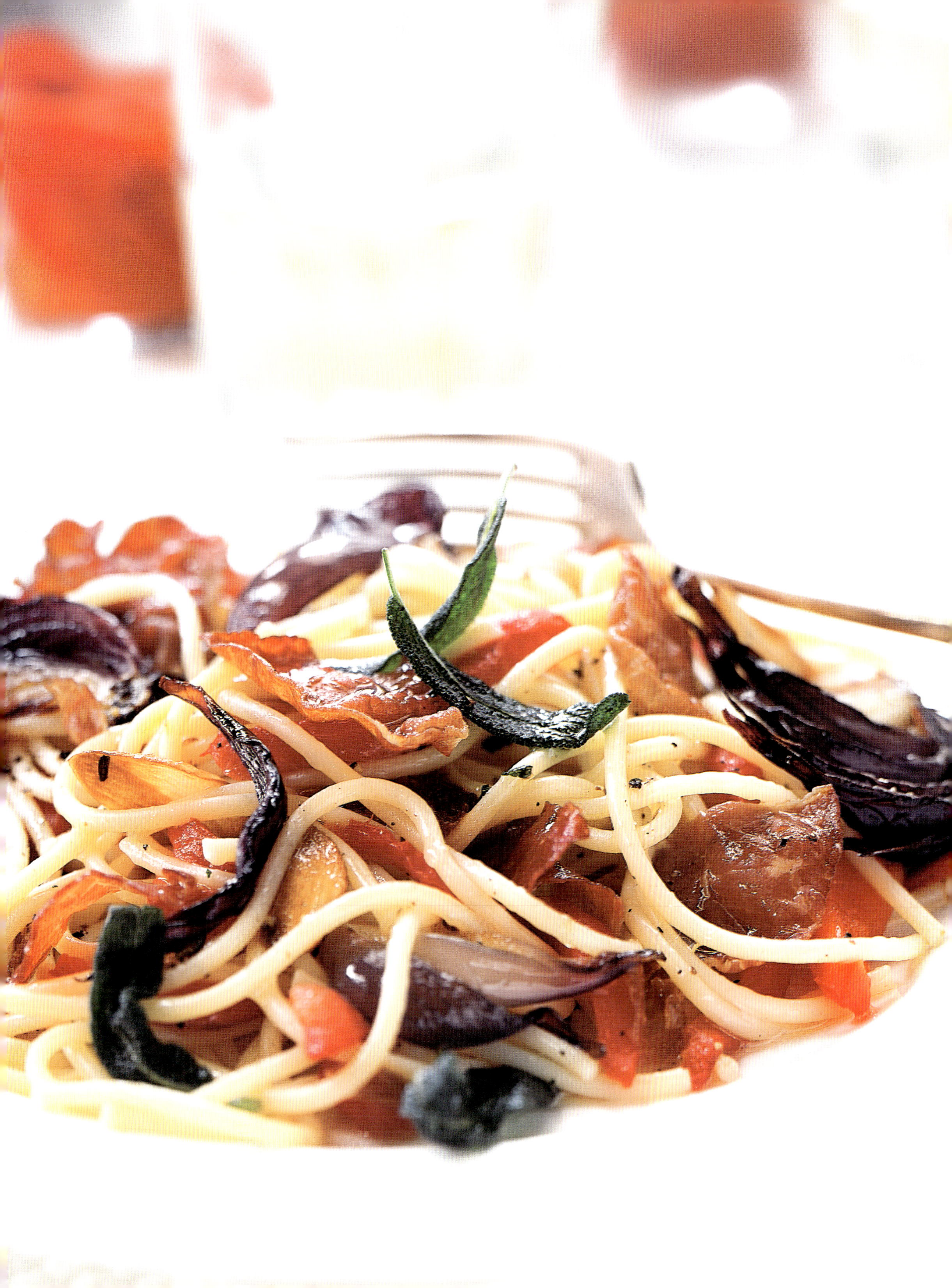

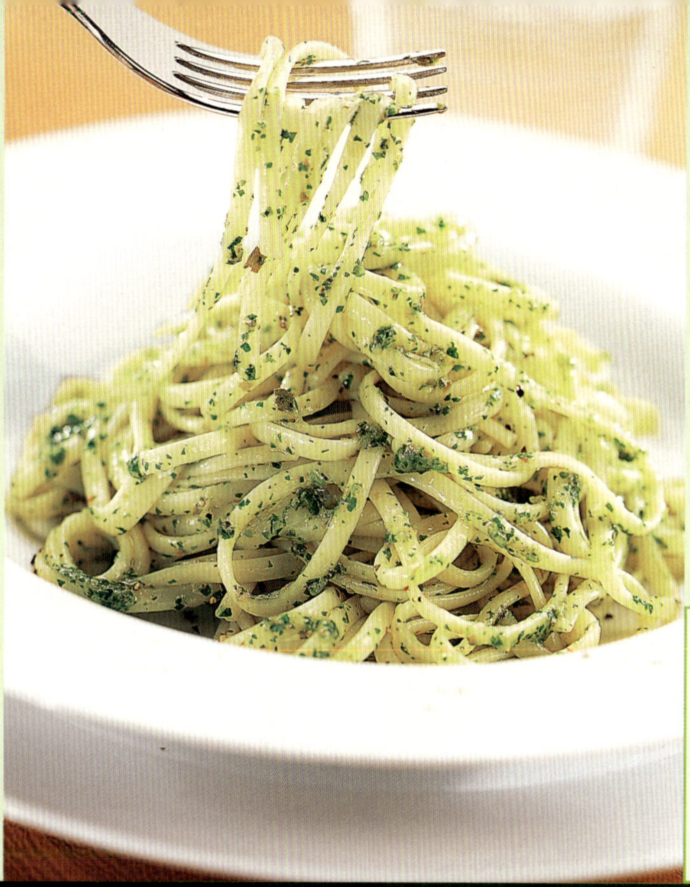

PER SERVING
269 kcalories
protein 7g
carbohydrate 34g
fat 13g
saturated fat 2g
fibre 2g
added sugar none
salt 0.79g

# Carbohydrates – the better half of a balanced diet

*We hear and use the term 'carbohydrates' so often that we all think we know exactly what they are... but are we entirely sure...? And why, as with cholesterol, do there seem to be 'good' and 'bad'?*

**What exactly are carbohydrates and why do we need them?**

*The simplest carbohydrates are sugars (monosaccharides, such as glucose and fructose, and disaccharides, such as sucrose and lactose, the naturally occurring sugar in milk). When these basic units are joined together in long chains or branching structures, they form polysaccharides or complex carbohydrates, such as starch and fibre. Starch comes from foods of plant origin, like rice and other grains, potatoes, pasta and bread. As sugar and starch, carbohydrates form a major energy-providing part of the human diet.*

**So are there 'bad' carbohydrates?**

*The simple sugars, once refined (table sugar, honey, etc.), no longer form part of the cellular structure of the food. Apart from supplying energy (i.e. calories) these 'extrinsic' or 'free' sugars, therefore, have none of the other benefits of carbohydrates, like fibre. They are also stripped of most of the vitamins, minerals and phytochemicals in the original plant. The 'intrinsic' sugars that naturally sweeten fruits and vegetables are much healthier in these respects. Because refined sugars are such potent suppliers of calories, their consumption also makes it much more difficult to get the right proportion of your calories in valuable nutritious forms. Most experts agree that it is our increased consumption of high-fat and highly refined sugar foods, such as cakes, biscuits, chocolate bars, etc., that has fuelled the growth in obesity.*

**How much carbohydrate do we need?**

*The World Health Organization recommends that we should get at least 50% of our calorie requirements in the form of complex carbohydrates and 'intrinsic' sugars – i.e. cereals, grains, pulses, vegetables and fruits. The Department of Health further recommends that only 10% of our calories are in the form of extrinsic sugars – which could be found in as little as 2 sweetened cups of tea and 3 or 4 chocolate biscuits a day!*

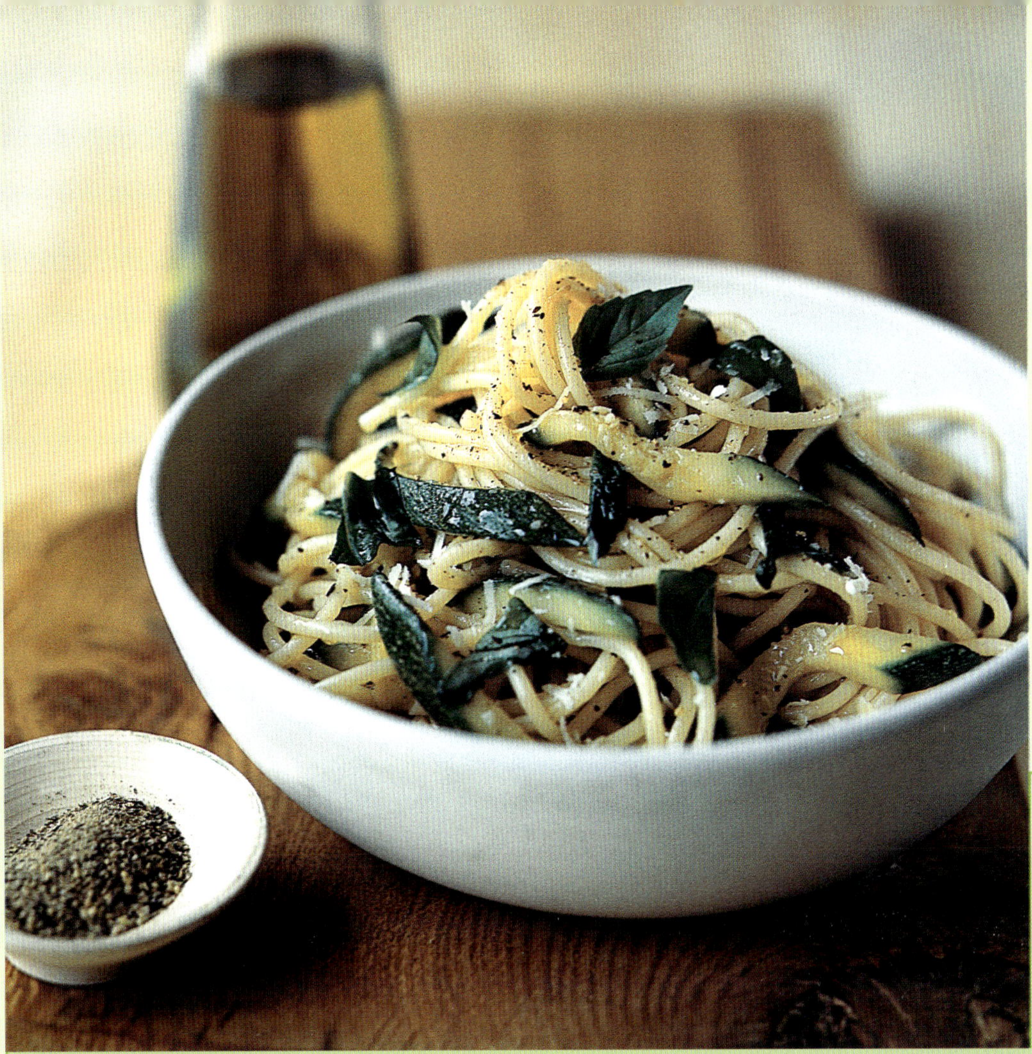

**PER SERVING**
466 kcalories
protein 19g
carbohydrate 65g
fat 16g
saturated fat 7g
fibre 4g
added sugar none
salt 0.75g

**Pasta is an ideal source of low-cost, low-fat complex carbohydrates ▼**

**Linguine with Watercress Sauce** *(opposite) needs 275g/10oz linguine or spaghetti cooked in a large pan of boiling salted water until tender but still firm to the bite. While the pasta cooks, put 1 garlic clove, 6 anchovies in oil, drained, and 1 tablespoon drained and well-rinsed capers in a food processor and process until well blended. Add 60g/2oz watercress and blend again until the mixture is finely chopped. With the motor still running, drizzle in 4 tablespoons olive oil to make a soft paste.*

*Mix 4 tablespoons of the pasta cooking water into the watercress sauce, then season to taste. Quickly drain the pasta and return to the pan. Stir in the sauce and divide between bowls. Grind over plenty of black pepper and serve immediately.*

**Spaghetti with Courgettes** *(above) comes from the Amalfi coast, where it was developed to provide instant nourishment for the fishermen after a stormy time at sea. To serve 6 generously: heat 3 tablespoons oil in a large frying pan. Season 1kg/2¼lb small courgettes, washed and cut into sticks, and cook gently for 3–4 minutes, stirring occasionally.*

*Cook 500g/1lb 2oz good-quality spaghetti in a large pan of boiling well salted water for 10–12 minutes, trying a strand of pasta every so often, and drain quickly while it is still al dente – tender but still firm to the bite. Turn the spaghetti into a large warmed serving bowl and stir in 85g/3oz freshly grated Parmesan, 30g/1oz butter and the courgettes. (It helps to have someone else adding the courgettes while you are lifting the pasta with a couple of forks.) Stir in 12 roughly torn basil leaves and add some more freshly ground black pepper. Serve immediately.*

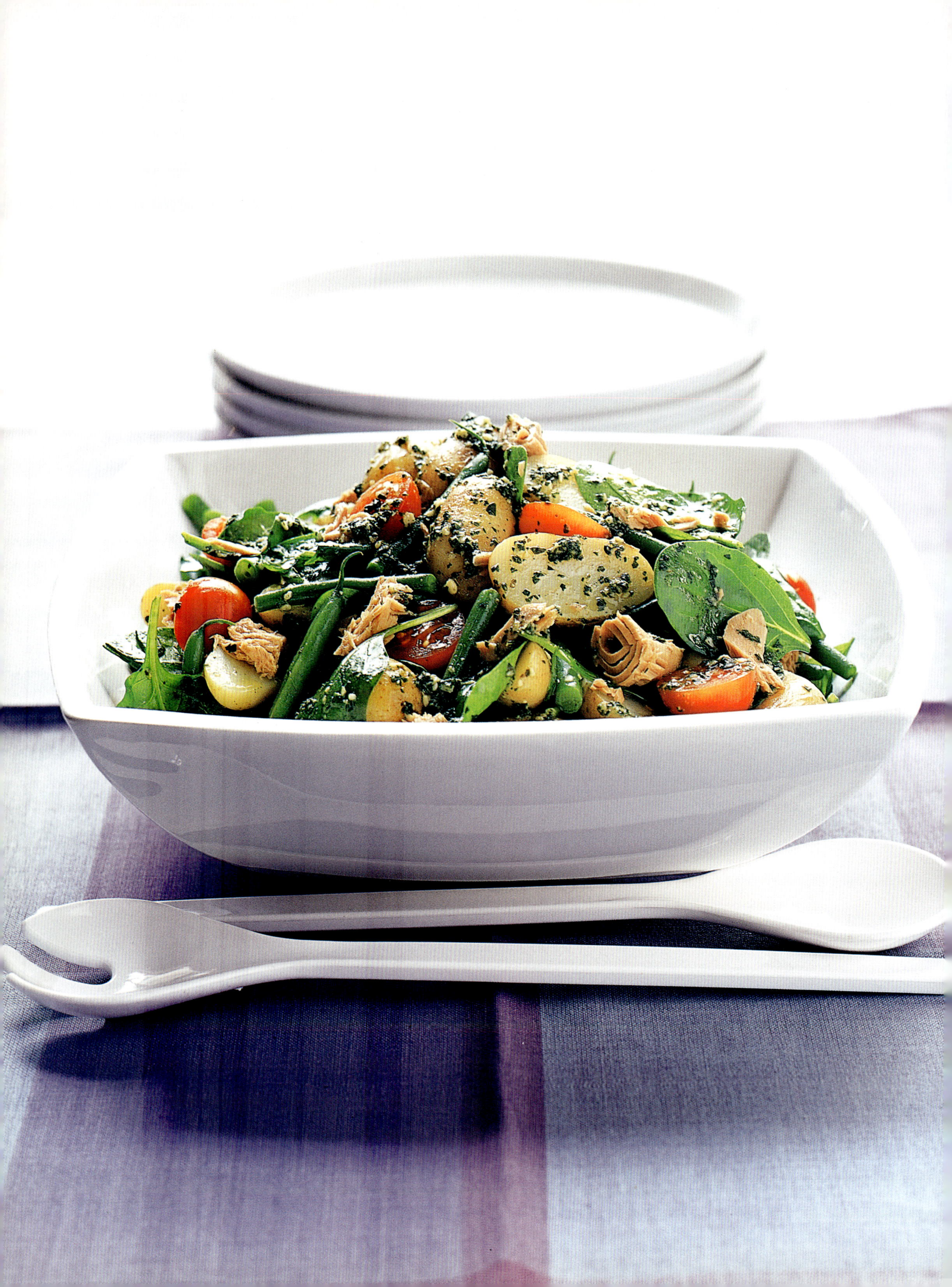

# Warm Potato and Tuna Salad with Pesto Dressing

**Although you may be tempted to buy tuna canned in brine, because it is lower in calories, packing in oil helps it preserve much more of its beneficial omega-3 oils.**

PER SERVING
**336 kcalories**
**protein 15g**
**carbohydrate 28g**
**fat 19g**
**saturated fat 3g**
**fibre 3g**
**added sugar none**
**salt 0.45g**

PREPARATION about 15 minutes
COOKING about 10 minutes

675g/1½lb new potatoes, halved lengthwise if large
225g/8oz green beans, halved
2 tbsp pesto (fresh is best)
4 tbsp olive oil
8 cherry tomatoes
175g/6oz can of tuna in oil, drained
couple of handfuls of spinach (preferably baby leaves, tear if larger)

1 Put the potatoes in a pan of boiling salted water, bring back to the boil and simmer for 8–10 minutes, adding the beans to the potatoes for about the last 3 minutes of cooking time.
2 Meanwhile, mix together the pesto and oil. Halve the tomatoes, drain and flake the tuna.
3 Drain the potatoes and beans and tip into a salad bowl. Stir in the spinach so it wilts a little in the warmth of the vegetables. Season. Scatter over the tomatoes and tuna, drizzle over the pesto and toss together.

# Creamy Broccoli and Mushroom Pasta

PER SERVING
**529 kcalories**
**protein 17g**
**carbohydrate 73g**
**fat 24g**
**saturated fat 5g**
**fibre 3g**
**added sugar 1g**
**salt 0.68g**

PREPARATION about 15 minutes
COOKING 10–12 minutes

350g/12oz farfalle or other pasta shape
250g/9oz broccoli, broken into small florets
1 tbsp olive oil
1 onion, finely chopped
250g/9oz chestnut mushrooms, sliced
200ml/7fl oz carton of crème fraîche
1 tbsp wholegrain mustard

1 Tip the pasta into a large pan of boiling water, stir well, then cook at a rolling boil for 10–12 minutes until just tender but still firm to the bite. Add the broccoli for the last 3 minutes of cooking.
2 Meanwhile, heat the oil in a frying pan and cook the onion for 8 minutes until softened and beginning to brown. Stir in the mushrooms and cook for 5 minutes more until tender. Stir in the crème fraîche and mustard to make a sauce.
3 Drain the pasta and broccoli and return to the pan. Stir in the sauce and serve immediately.

# Courgette and Saffron Risotto

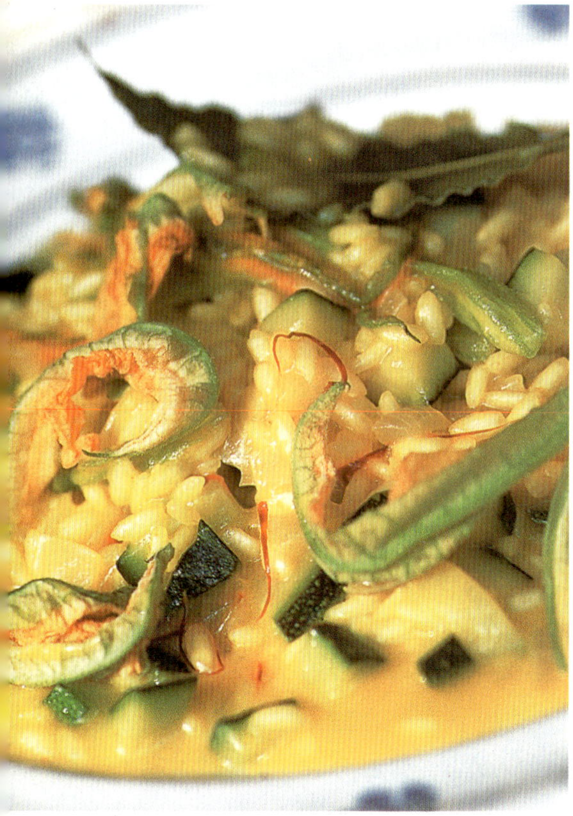

**Courgette flowers, once only found in trendy restaurants, are now creeping into some supermarkets.**

SERVES 6 as a starter or 4 as a main course
PREPARATION 15 minutes
COOKING 30 minutes

1.3 litres/2¼ pints vegetable stock
45g/1½oz butter
2 tbsp olive oil
1 large onion, finely chopped
2 bay leaves
2 courgettes (with flowers if possible), any flowers detached and the courgettes diced
350g/12oz risotto rice
large pinch of saffron strands
150ml/¼ pint dry white wine
30g/1oz freshly grated Parmesan, plus more for sprinkling

PER SERVING (for 6)
**344 kcalories • protein 8g • carbohydrate 49g fat 12g • saturated fat 6g • fibre 2g added sugar none • salt 1.26g**

1 Bring the stock to a simmer in a pan. Meanwhile, melt 30g/1oz of the butter with the oil in a large, heavy-based pan, then cook the onions with the bay leaves over a moderate heat, stirring frequently.
2 When the onion is softened, stir in the diced courgettes and cook for 1 minute, then stir in the rice. After 10 minutes, stir in the saffron and courgette flowers, each torn into 4 or 5 pieces. Add the wine and cook, stirring, until the wine has been absorbed.
3 Add the stock and finish cooking as in the recipe below.

# Wild Mushroom Risotto

PER SERVING
**482 kcalories**
**protein 13g**
**carbohydrate 64g**
**fat 19g**
**saturated fat 9g**
**fibre 2g**
**added sugar none**
**salt 1.34g**

**This makes a luscious starter for a dinner party, especially for vegetarians.**

PREPARATION 30 minutes, plus 20 minutes' soaking
COOKING 40 minutes

30g/1oz dried porcini, or a mixture of dried wild mushrooms
1 litre/1¾ pints chicken or vegetable stock
45g/1½oz butter
2 tbsp olive oil
2 tbsp finely chopped shallots
225g/8oz firm cultivated white or chestnut mushrooms, cubed if large or sliced if small
300g/10oz risotto rice, such as Arborio
125ml/4fl oz dry white wine
30g/1oz freshly grated Parmesan, plus more for sprinkling

1 Put the dried mushrooms in a bowl, add enough stock to cover and soak for 20 minutes. Strain the liquid into the remaining stock. Coarsely chop the soaked mushrooms.
2 Bring the stock to a simmer in a pan. Meanwhile, melt 30g/1oz butter with the oil in a large, heavy pan, then cook the shallots with all the mushrooms over a moderate heat, stirring frequently, until the mushrooms have reabsorbed any liquid they give off. Add the rice and stir to coat. Add the wine and cook, stirring, until absorbed.
3 Add the stock a ladleful at a time, stirring over a gentle heat for about 20 minutes until the rice is almost tender. Perfect risotto is creamy but not solid, and the rice should still have a little bite. If the rice is particularly absorbent and the stock is used before it is tender, add boiling water.
4 Remove from the heat, beat in the remaining butter and the grated Parmesan; season with salt and pepper to taste. Cover and leave to stand for about a minute before serving on warm plates, sprinkled with more grated Parmesan.

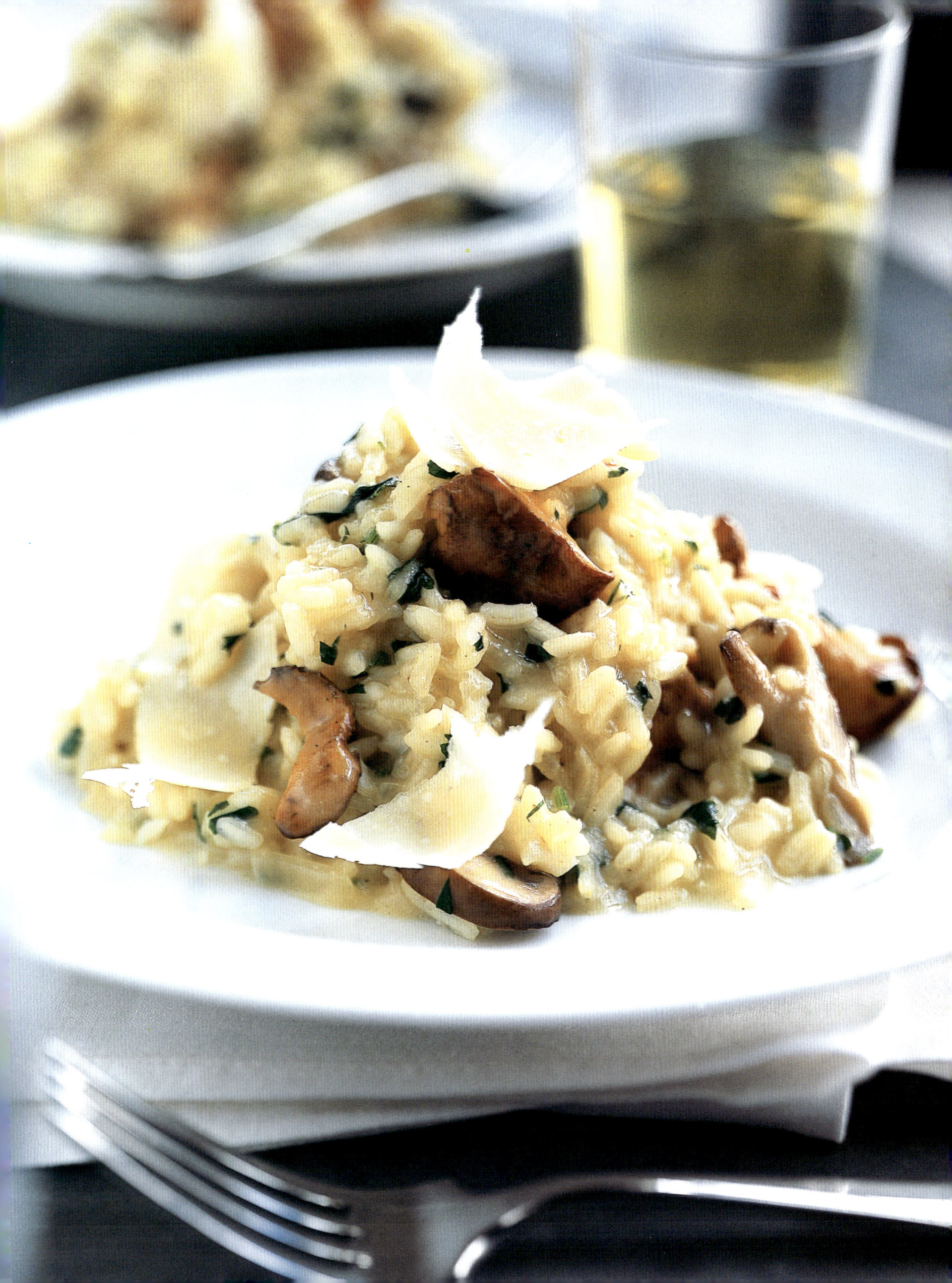

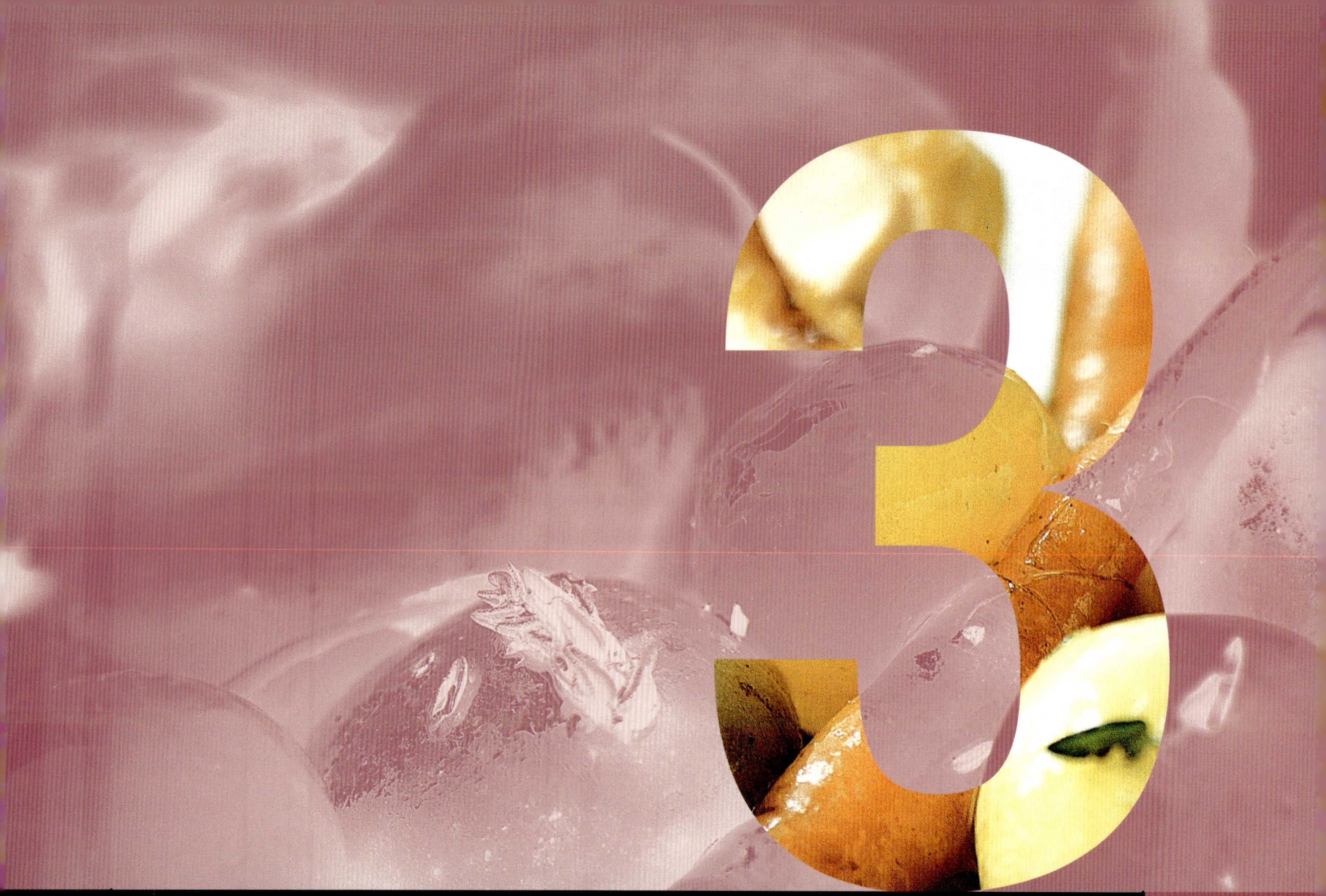

3

# Fit Family Meals

*Perhaps the greatest challenge – and the greatest concern – is turning out food on a regular basis that will not only satisfy the family but provide them with a healthy balanced diet. Children and teenagers may turn up their noses at plainly cooked vegetables, but there are ways of building these – and other healthy ingredients – into a wide range of dishes, including the sorts of things that young people love, like pizza. Even basic staples like potatoes and rice can be given makeovers to provide them with new interest and added nutritive value.*

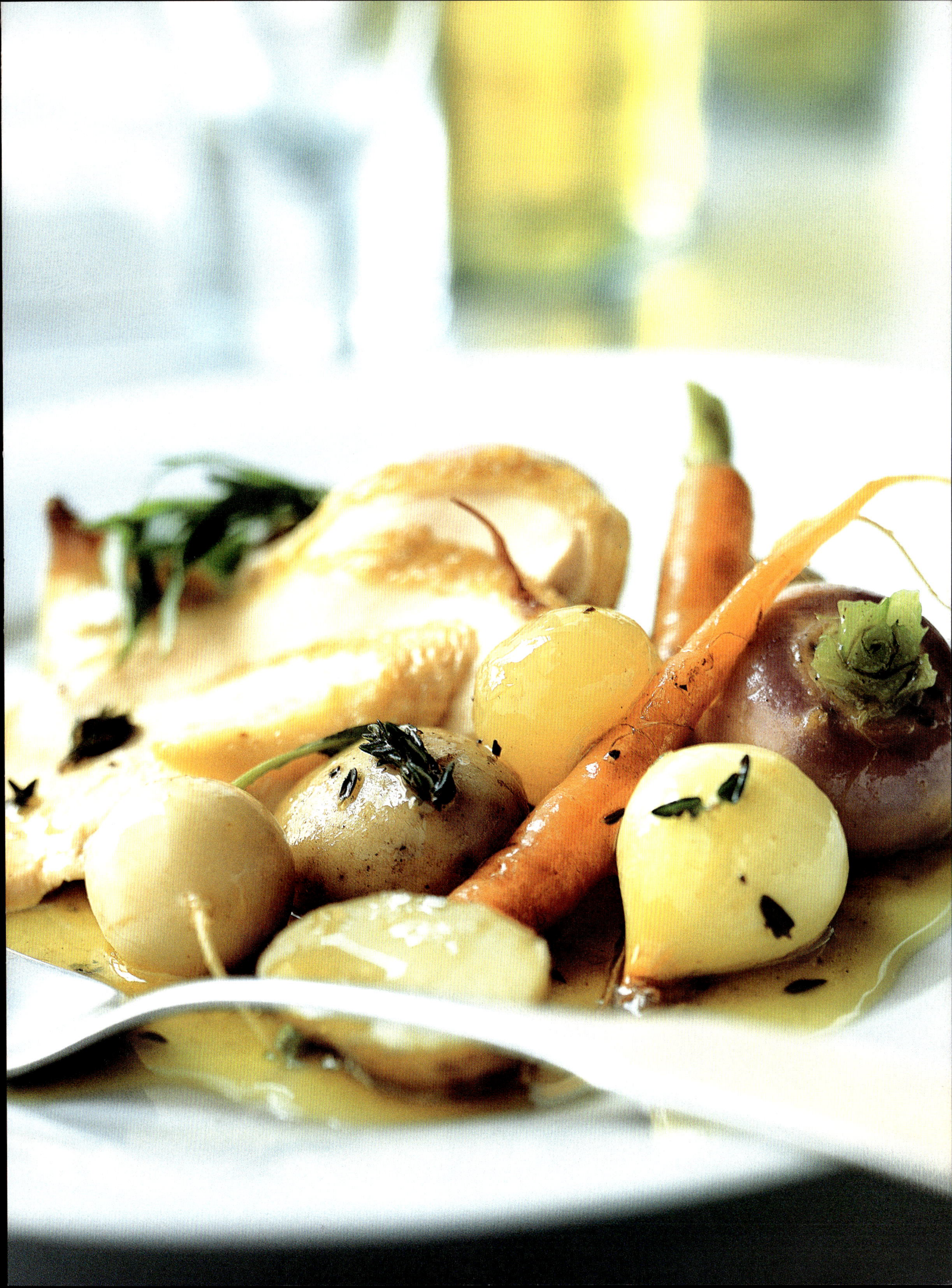

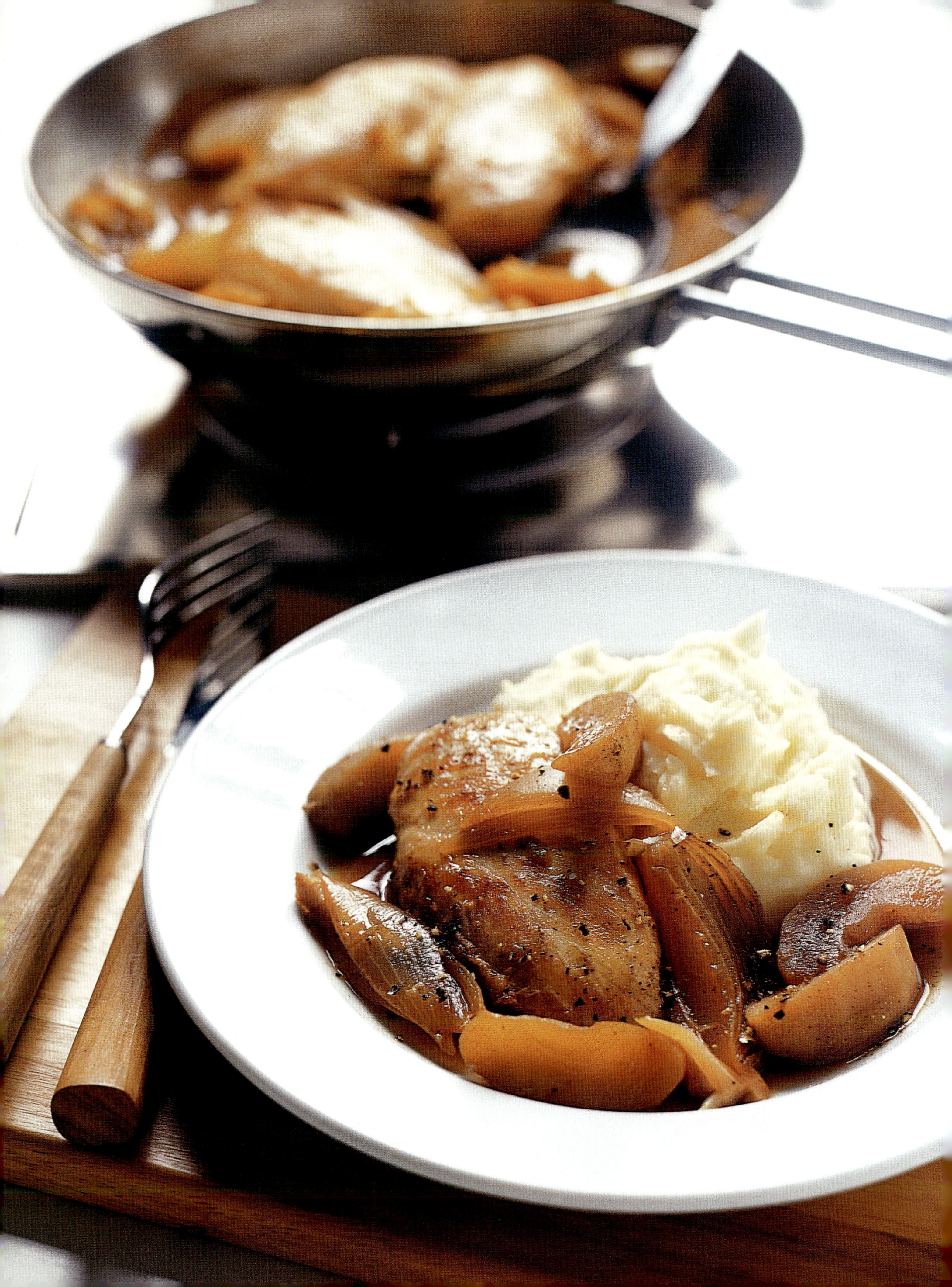

# Lemon and Herb Chicken in a Pot

PER SERVING
636 kcalories
protein 44g
carbohydrate 27g
fat 40g
saturated fat 2g
fibre 5g
added sugar none
salt 1.54g

**Use an unwaxed lemon if you can find one, or scrub an ordinary one thoroughly before you pare the rind, as ordinary lemons are coated in wax impregnated with a chemical cocktail to lengthen shelf-life. It's well worth spending a little extra on a plump corn-fed bird. They're usually tender, with yellowy skin and fat, and tasty – with none of that fish-meal flavour in the dark meat that you get from cheaper birds (because that's what they've been fed on). You can buy them from most supermarkets, or order one from your butcher. For less calories and fat, remove the chicken skin before serving.**

PREPARATION 15 minutes
COOKING about 1³/₄ hours

large knob of butter
1 tbsp olive oil
1 chicken, about 1.3–1.8kg/3–4lb, preferably corn-fed
225g/8oz shallots or small onions
850ml/1½ pints chicken stock
1 lemon
2–3 sprigs of fresh thyme, plus more to garnish
2–3 sprigs of fresh tarragon, plus more to garnish
225g/8oz baby turnips
225g/8oz baby carrots
450g/1lb small new potatoes

1 Preheat the oven to 190°C/375°F/Gas 5. Heat the butter and oil in a very large flameproof casserole. Add the chicken, breast-side down, and cook over a moderate heat for about 8 minutes, turning so the breast browns evenly. Remove the casserole from the heat and turn the chicken the right way up. Add the shallots or onions, pour in the stock, then return to the heat and bring to simmering point. Season to taste.
2 Using a potato peeler or small sharp knife, pare the rind thinly from the lemon; squeeze the juice. Add the rind and juice to the casserole with the thyme and tarragon sprigs. Cover and cook in the oven for 45 minutes.
3 Remove the casserole from the oven and add the turnips, carrots and potatoes. Return to the oven for a further 45 minutes until the vegetables are tender. Check the chicken is done by piercing the thickest part with a skewer – if the juices run clear, it is cooked. Discard the strips of rind and adjust the seasoning of the vegetables.
4 Lift the chicken on to a board and carve. Put some chicken and vegetables on plates, ladle over some of the stock and garnish with thyme and tarragon sprigs. (Cool any remaining stock quickly, then cover and chill or freeze; use as stock for soup.)

# Chicken with Apples and Cider

PER SERVING
269 kcalories
protein 34g
carbohydrate 12g
fat 7g
saturated fat 1g
fibre 2g
added sugar none
salt 0.36g

PREPARATION about 10 minutes
COOKING about 25 minutes

2 tbsp oil
4 skinless chicken breast fillets
1 onion, cut into wedges
2 eating apples, such as Cox's, peeled, cored and each cut into 8 wedges
300ml/½ pint dry cider
150ml/¼ pint chicken stock
rice or mashed potato, to serve

1 Heat the oil in a large frying pan and fry the chicken breasts for 3–4 minutes on each side until golden. Remove from the pan and set aside.
2 Lower the heat slightly and add the onion. Fry, stirring, for 2–3 minutes until tinged brown. Add the apple and cook over a high heat for 5 minutes until golden.
3 Still over a high heat, pour in the cider and bubble for 2 minutes to reduce slightly. Add the stock, stirring to scrape the bits from the bottom of the pan. Lower the heat.
4 Return the chicken to the pan, cover and simmer for 5 minutes until it is almost cooked. Remove the lid and simmer for 3–4 minutes to thicken the sauce a little. Season and serve with rice or mashed potato.

# Quick Chicken Satay

PER SERVING
249 kcalories
protein 29g
carbohydrate 3g
fat 14g
saturated fat 2g
fibre 1g
added sugar 1g
salt 0.34g

**This way with chicken avoids oily marinades, sauces or dips and can obviously be made even lower in fat by removing the chicken skin. The peanut butter used in the satay sauce is a good source of lots of nutrients, including the B vitamins and antioxidant vitamin E.**

PREPARATION 10 minutes
COOKING 25 minutes

4 chicken breast fillets
about 1 tsp chilli powder
juice of about 3 lemons (you need 6 tbsp)
3 tbsp good-quality crunchy peanut butter
1 tsp sugar

1 Preheat the grill or barbecue. To grill, line a grill pan with foil, then lay the chicken on it. Sprinkle with some chilli, 1 tablespoon of lemon juice, then season. To barbecue, put the chicken in a dish and sprinkle with the chilli, lemon juice and seasoning. Transfer to the grill or barbecue and cook for 25 minutes, turning, until cooked through.
2 To make the satay sauce: put the peanut butter, sugar and half a teaspoon of chilli powder in a bowl and mix together. Gradually beat in the remaining lemon juice.
3 Serve each chicken breast with a spoonful of satay sauce.

# Thai Chicken and Coconut Curry

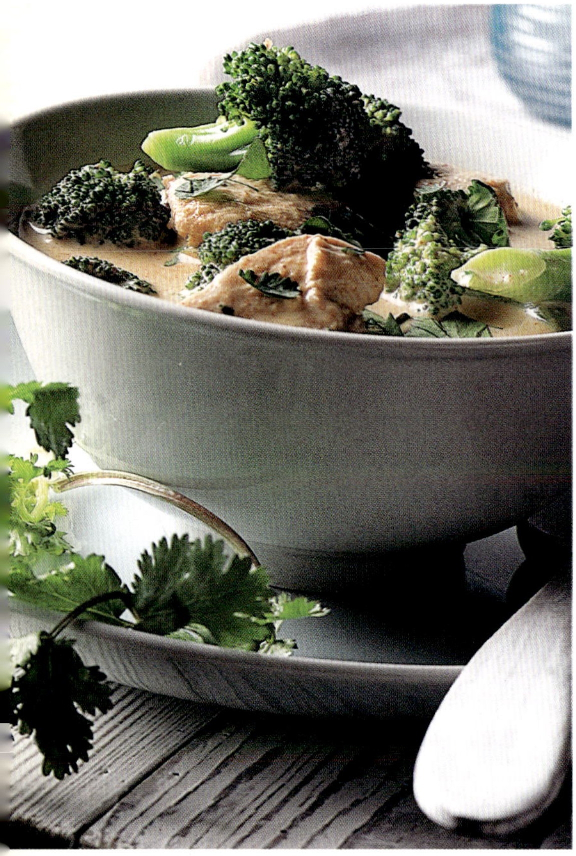

**Coconuts are unusual in the vegetable world for their high percentage of saturated fats. Some research, however, shows that these don't have quite the same adverse effect on the body as animal saturates. If you want to reduce the fat content, replace the coconut cream with thick low-fat yoghurt (don't let it boil) and impart coconut flavour by stirring a spoonful of coconut cream as you serve.**

PREPARATION about 10 minutes
COOKING 12–15 minutes

1–2 tbsp red Thai curry paste
450g/1lb skinless chicken breast fillets, cut into bite-sized cubes
225g/8oz broccoli florets
200ml/7fl oz coconut cream
good handful of fresh coriander

PER SERVING
336 kcalories
protein 29g
carbohydrate 4g
fat 23g
saturated fat 16g
fibre 3g
added sugar none
salt 0.42g

1 Blend the curry paste in a small bowl with 2 tablespoons of water, then pour into a pan. Add the chicken with some seasoning and 150ml/$^1/_4$ pint water. Bring to the boil. Lower the heat, cover tightly and cook for 12–15 minutes, until just tender.
2 While the chicken is cooking, cook the broccoli in boiling salted water for 5 minutes until just tender. Drain and stir into the chicken with the coconut cream. Bring to a gentle simmer then cook, covered, for 2–3 minutes.
3 Chop the coriander roughly (save some leaves for garnishing) and stir into the curry. Serve with Thai or long-grain rice, and garnished with the reserved coriander leaves.

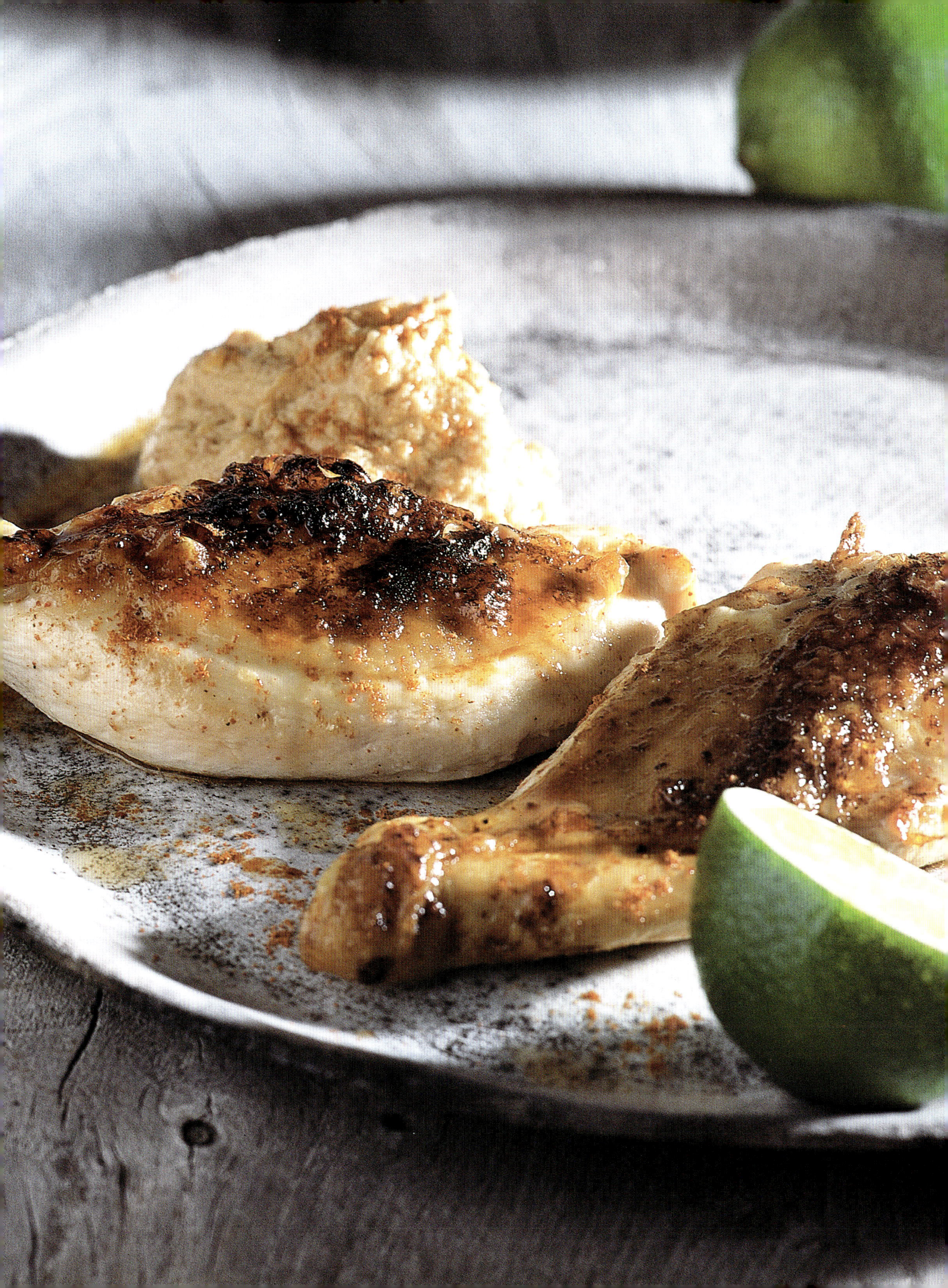

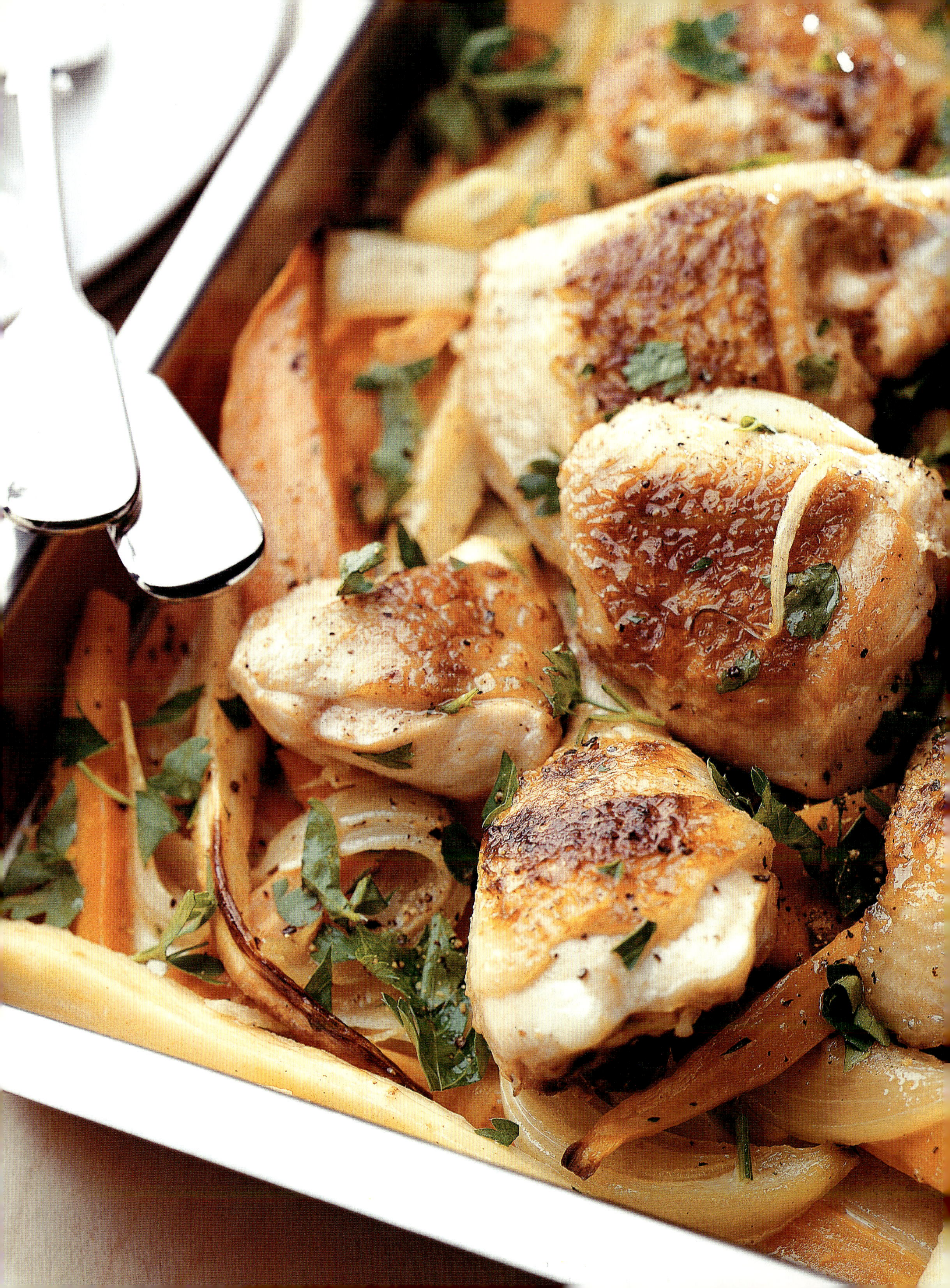

# Braised Winter Chicken and Vegetables

PER SERVING
415 kcalories
protein 26g
carbohydrate 32g
fat 21g
saturated fat 9g
fibre 8g
added sugar none
salt 0.87g

PREPARATION
about 20 minutes
COOKING
about 40 minutes

**If you are concerned about fat and/or calorie intake, skin the chicken pieces and don't add any cream.**

2 onions, each cut into 8 wedges
4 parsnips, cut into sticks
4 carrots, cut into sticks
1 sweet potato, cut into sticks
3 strips of lemon rind
450ml/¾ pint chicken stock
8 chicken pieces (mixture of thighs and drumsticks)
small bunch of fresh parsley, roughly chopped
4 tbsp crème fraîche or double cream

1 Preheat the oven to 190°C/375°F/Gas 5. Put all the vegetables and lemon rind in an ovenproof dish and pour over the stock. Put in the oven for 10 minutes.
2 Meanwhile, heat a dry non-stick frying pan, then brown the chicken pieces on all sides. Lay the chicken on the vegetables and season, then bake for about 25 minutes until the chicken is cooked (when you pierce the thickest part with the tip of a knife, the juices run clear).
3 Stir in the parsley and cream, and serve.

# Mediterranean Chicken Pasta

PER SERVING
624 kcalories
protein 33g
carbohydrate 74g
fat 24g
saturated fat 8g
fibre 4g
added sugar none
salt 1.12g

PREPARATION
about 20 minutes
COOKING
20 minutes

2 skinless chicken breast fillets, cut into chunks
1 red onion, cut into 8 wedges
1 red pepper, deseeded and cut into 8 strips
2 garlic cloves, unpeeled
3 tbsp olive oil
350g/12oz pasta, such as rigatoni
4 tbsp ready-made pesto
225g/8oz cherry tomatoes, halved
85g/3oz firm goats' cheese or feta

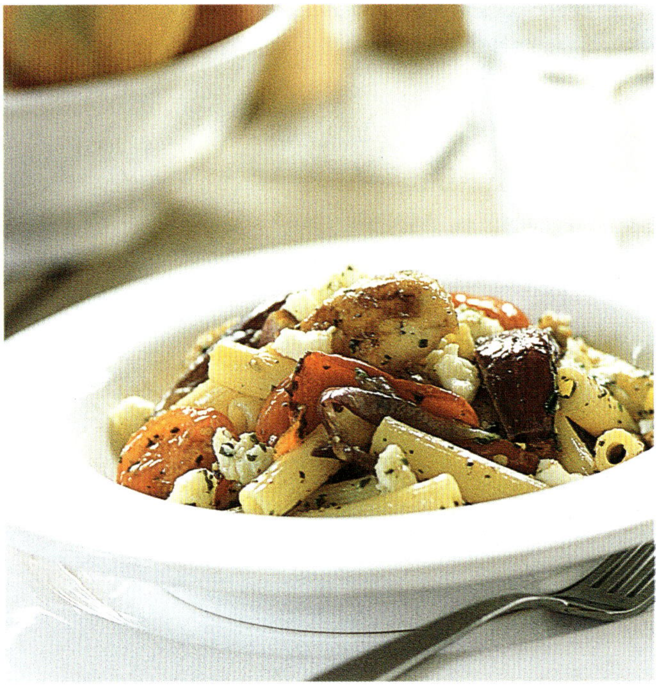

1 Preheat the oven to 200°C/400°F/Gas 6. Put the chicken, onion, red pepper and garlic cloves in a roasting tin and drizzle with the oil. Season and mix with a spoon to ensure everything is well coated in the oil. Roast for 20 minutes.
2 After the chicken has been cooking for 5 minutes, cook the pasta in a pan of boiling salted water until just tender but still firm to the bite. Drain well.
3 When the chicken and vegetables are cooked, remove them from the oven. Slip the garlic out of its skin and mash in the tin with a spoon. Tip in the pasta, pesto and tomatoes, and carefully mix together.
4 Crumble the cheese over the mixture, adjust the seasoning and serve.

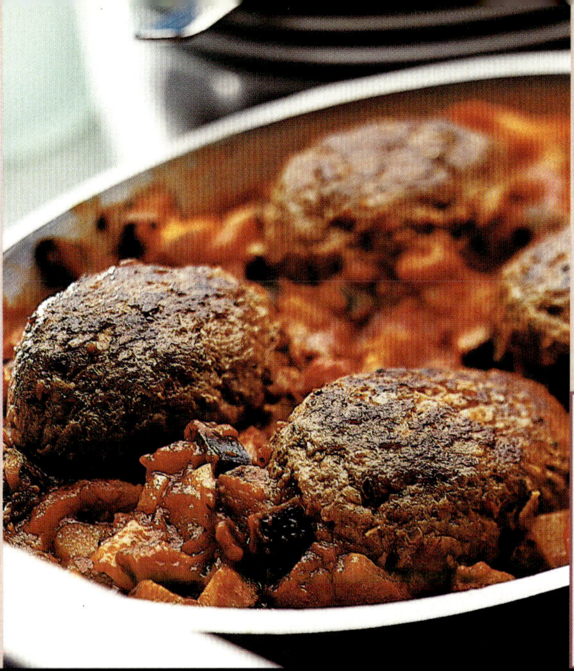

**PER SERVING**
271 kcalories
protein 34g
carbohydrate 16g
fat 9g
saturated fat 2g
fibre 6g
added sugar 1g
salt 0.76g

# Healthy food on a budget

*You quite often hear people say that eating healthily necessarily means spending more money. These are probably the same people who will happily spend three or four times as much for a convenience pack of ready-made mashed potatoes as make their own because they are used to 'low-calorie' and 'low-fat' versions of that sort of food being higher in price. The truth is quite different, however, as it is actually quite easy to eat well-balanced and healthy food – and save money!*

### What are the best things to spend limited resources on?

*Think of the way the rest of the world eats, outside the spoiled surfeit of the industrialized nations, and the answer to this is obvious. There is fantastic nutrition to be had from some of the humblest staples, like rice, oats, barley, pasta or noodles, lentils and all sorts of pulses. Also, the more whole the food is the more nutritive value it retains – it is truly the great paradox of human nutrition that the more processed and refined a food is the more expensive it obviously becomes but the less value it really has for us.*

### Surely getting my 'five a day' is going to be expensive?

*Obviously some fruit and veg can be expensive, but if you buy local produce in season, it will usually be fairly reasonable. Moreover, things like apples, bananas and oranges, tomatoes, onions, parsnips, carrots and cabbage (most of which are 'superfoods', see page 100) can be had at economical prices all year round.*

### What are the best things to save on?

*One of the most important things to remember in this context is that we all eat far too much of the type of food that usually costs the most – protein. Try to quash for once and for all the 'meat and two veg' mentality and think along more healthy Mediterranean lines of the protein element of a meal being more of a flavouring finishing touch than its basis. That way, say, a single piece of steak, thinly sliced, can feed 4 people as part of a tasty steak, mushroom and onion stroganoff on a bed of noodles, without anyone feeling that anything has in any way been skimped.*

*Remember that if you are getting enough of a good range of complex carbohydrates (see page 36) – like vegetables, pulses, grain, pasta, etc. – you are probably getting a good proportion of the protein you actually need from them – and excess protein is credited by some with all sorts of health problems. Of course, animal protein also tends to come with quite a high percentage of saturated fat – yet another very good reason to choose this as the ideal area in which to economize.*

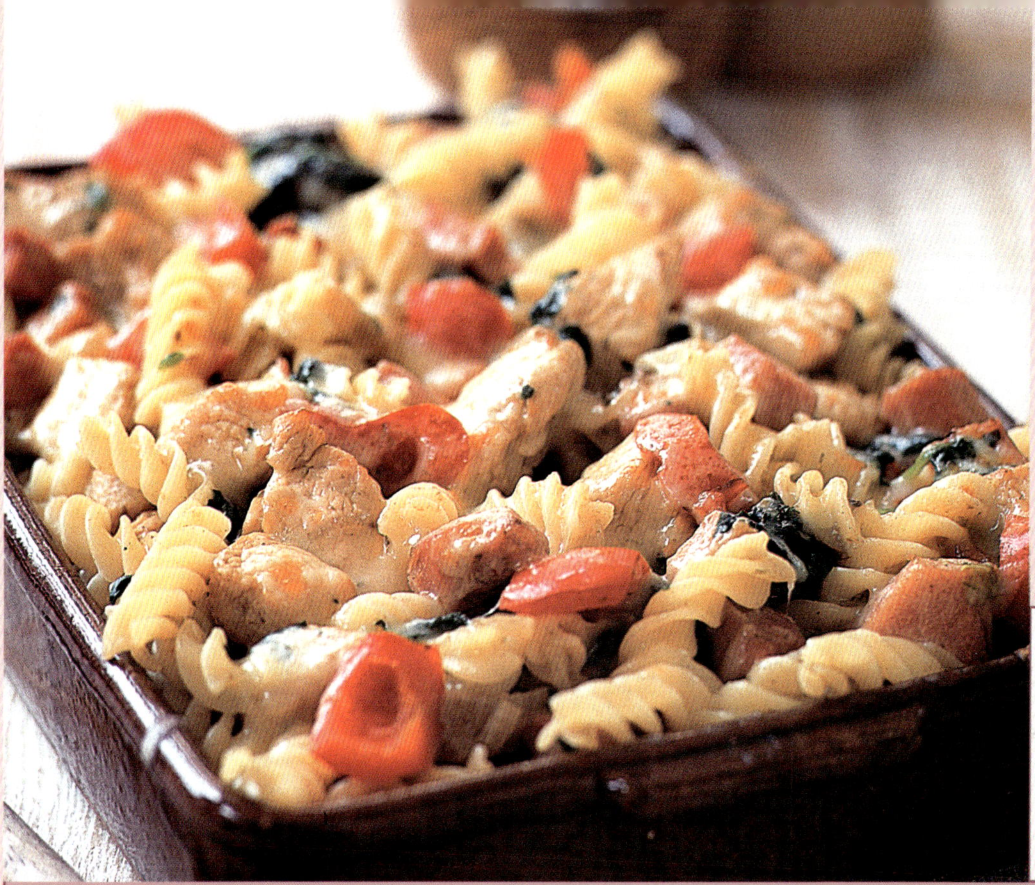

**PER SERVING**
509 kcalories
protein 39g
carbohydrate 58g
fat 15g
saturated fat 6g
fibre 4g
added sugar none
salt 1.5g

**For those with growing kids and/or who just can't wean themselves off meat, turkey is an excellent source of low-cost, low-fat protein ▼**

*Ratatouille Meatballs (opposite) are made by blending 1 garlic clove and 1 small onion in a food processor. Add 500g/1lb 2oz turkey mince and 1 teaspoon of dried oregano. Season and process until well blended. Shape into 4 large balls and flatten slightly. Heat a tablespoon of oil in a frying pan and cook the meatballs for 8–10 minutes, turning, until browned all over. Put on a plate.*

*Heat another tablespoon of oil in the pan and fry a chopped garlic clove and second small onion with another teaspoon of dried oregano, 2 diced courgettes, 1 diced aubergine and 1 deseeded and diced yellow pepper for 5 minutes. Add two 400g/14oz cans of plum tomatoes, 2 tablespoons tomato purée, 1/2 teaspoon sugar and 2 teaspoons Worcestershire sauce. Bring to the boil, add the meatballs, cover and simmer for 30 minutes. Serve with crusty bread.*

*Turkey and Mushroom Fusilli (above) is perfect for an inexpensive special family supper for 6. Heat 1 tablespoon olive oil in a large pan, then cook the 1 sliced onion and 1 deseeded and chopped red pepper for 5 minutes. Add 450g/1lb turkey fillet, cut into chunks, and cook for another 5 minutes, stirring occasionally.*

*Cook 350g/12oz fusilli pasta in a pan of boiling salted water for about 8–10 minutes until just tender but still firm to the bite. Drain well. Preheat the grill to hot.*

*Add to the turkey in the pan a 300g–350g/10–12 oz carton of mushroom sauce (or a can of condensed mushroom soup if on a really tight budget; alternatively, should you want to push the boat out slightly, you could use wild mushroom sauce for a really deep flavour), made up to 600ml/1 pint with milk. Bring to the boil. Stir in the drained pasta, 100g/4oz sliced ham, cut into chunks and 225g/8oz frozen leaf spinach. Season and add freshly grated nutmeg to taste. Simmer for 5 minutes until piping hot. Spoon into a shallow heatproof dish, sprinkle with 85g/3oz grated mature Cheddar cheese and grill until brown.*

# Meal-in-a-bowl Noodle Soup

**Noodles are becoming increasingly popular, and the real things are so easy and convenient. Look for fresh Japanese udon or yakisoba noodles in the ethnic section of the supermarket.**

SERVES 1 (easily doubled)
PREPARATION about 10 minutes
COOKING 8 minutes

1 tsp vegetable oil
4–5 mushrooms, sliced
1 garlic clove, finely chopped
½ red pepper, deseeded and cut into strips
1 small stalk of broccoli, broken into florets
211g/7½oz pack fresh soupy udon or yakisoba noodles
300ml/½ pint boiling water

1 Heat the oil in a medium pan. Add the mushrooms, garlic, red pepper and broccoli and stir-fry until the vegetables are beginning to soften, about 4 minutes.
2 Stir in the contents of the flavouring sachet from the noodle pack and pour over the boiling water. Add the noodles and cook for 2 minutes until just tender and boiling hot.

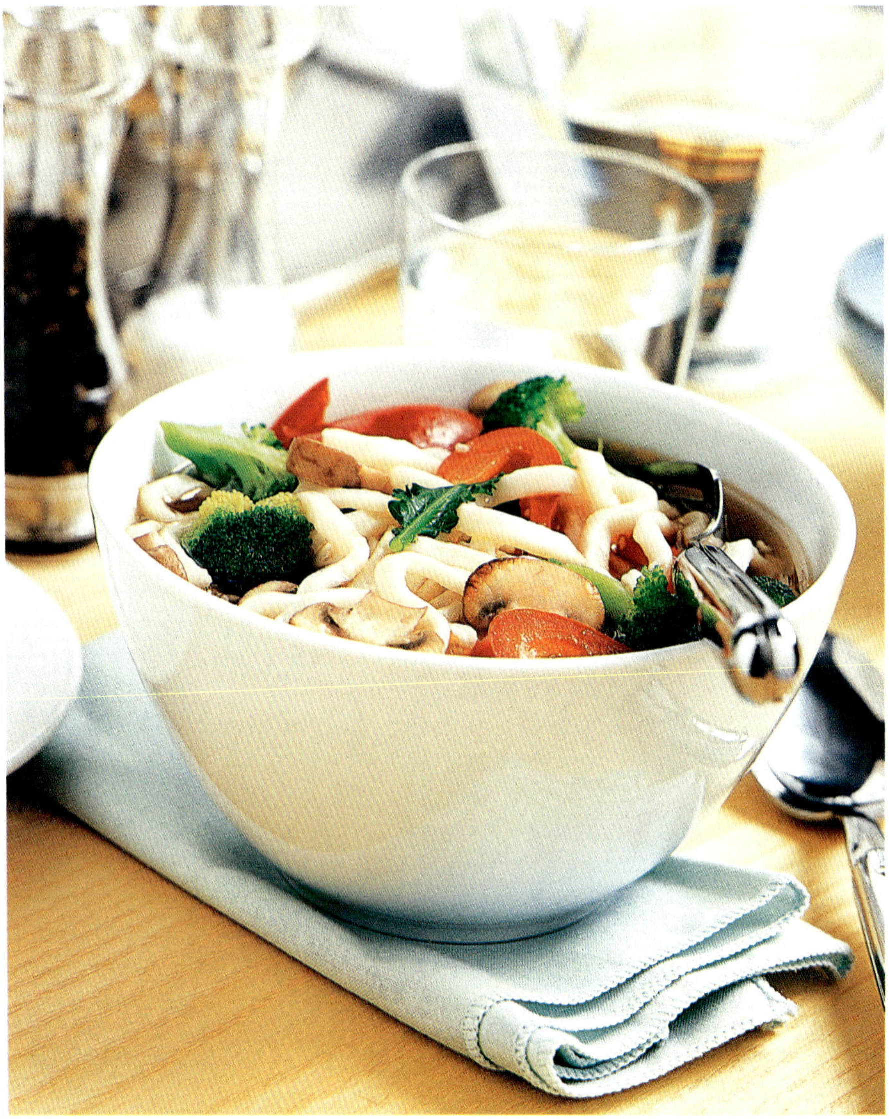

PER SERVING
**457 kcalories**
**protein 16g**
**carbohydrate 84g**
**fat 9g**
**saturated fat 0.2g**
**fibre 5g**
**added sugar none**
**salt 0.02g**

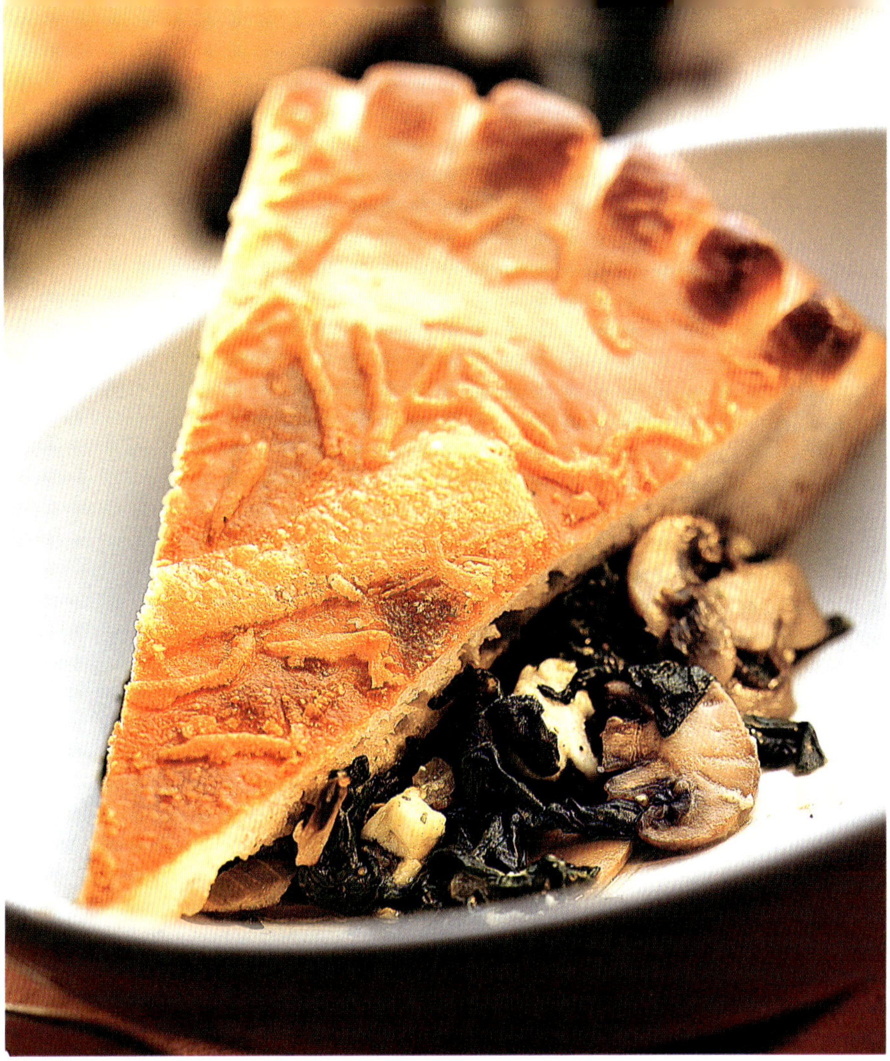

PER SERVING
672 kcalories
protein 31g
carbohydrate 88g
fat 22g
saturated fat 9g
fibre 7g
added sugar 3g
salt 3.86g

# Spinach and Feta Pizza Pie

PREPARATION 20 minutes
COOKING 30–35 minutes

500g/1lb 2oz frozen leaf spinach, defrosted
1 tbsp oil, plus more for brushing
1 onion, chopped
150g/5oz mushrooms, sliced
175g/6oz feta cheese, crumbled
4 tbsp freshly grated Parmesan cheese
1 egg, beaten
290g/10 oz packet of bread mix
tomato and red onion salad, to serve

**There is a whole range of delicious healthy toppings/fillings for pizza: try blanched broccoli florets and chopped anchovy fillets; sliced courgettes with masses of fresh basil or flaked tuna; red onion wedges, seedless raisins and pine nuts; or fresh sardines with black olives.**

1 Preheat the oven to 200°C/400°F/Gas 6. Tip the spinach into a colander and press with the back of a wooden spoon to extract as much water as possible. Transfer to a large bowl.
2 Heat the oil in a pan and fry the onion until softened (about 5 minutes), then add the mushrooms and fry briefly. Tip into the bowl of spinach, then add the feta, 3 tablespoons of the grated Parmesan and most of the beaten egg. Season with salt and pepper (carefully, as the feta is already very salty). Mix well.
3 Make the bread mix according to the packet instructions. Roll out half of the dough into a 30cm/12in round and transfer to an oiled baking sheet. Spread with the spinach and feta filling to within a finger's width of the edge. Brush the edge of the dough with the remaining beaten egg. Roll out the remaining dough and use to cover the pie, pinching the edges to seal in the filling.
4 Brush the top of the pie with a little oil and sprinkle with the remaining Parmesan. Bake for 25–30 minutes until crisp and golden.
5 Serve warm, cut into wedges, with a tomato and red onion salad.

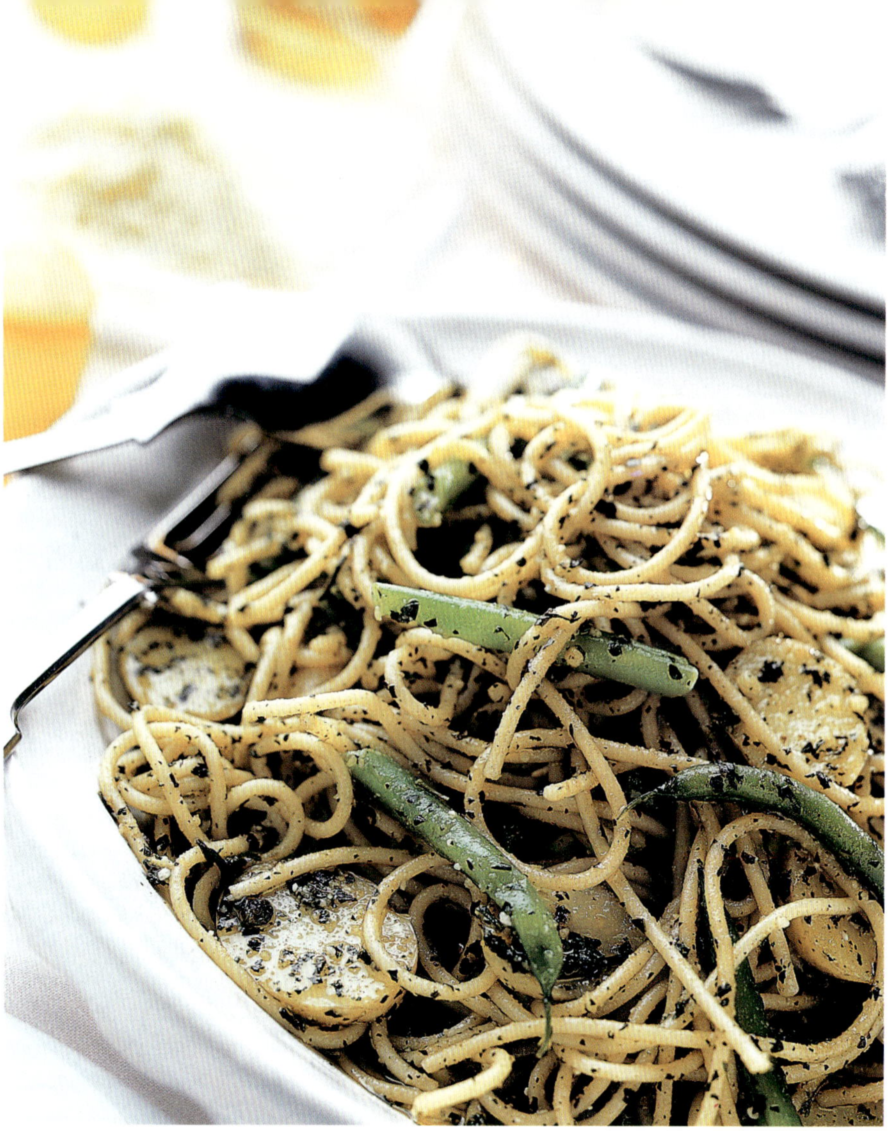

**PER SERVING**
**416 kcalories**
**protein 13g**
**carbohydrate 70g**
**fat 12g**
**saturated fat 4g**
**fibre 4g**
**added sugar none**
**salt 0.21g**

# Spaghetti Genovese

**It's worth hunting out tubs of fresh pesto (you'll need about half a tub - use the rest to dress plain pasta or to zip up some minestrone) as they have a livelier flavour and are a more appetizing shade of green than pesto in jars. They are stocked in chiller cabinets in larger supermarkets.**

PREPARATION 10 minutes
COOKING 20 minutes

300g/10oz new potatoes, cubed
300g/10oz spaghetti
225g/8oz green beans, cut in half
60g/2oz fresh pesto
olive oil, for drizzling

1 Pour boiling water into a very large pan until half full. Bring back to the boil, then add the potatoes and spaghetti with a little salt. Cook for 15 minutes until the potatoes and pasta are tender and the potatoes just keep their shape, adding the green beans just for the last 5 minutes of cooking time. Drain well, reserving 4 tablespoons of the cooking liquid.
2 Return the potatoes, pasta and beans to the pan and stir in the fresh pesto and reserved cooking liquid. Season to taste, then divide between 4 serving plates and drizzle with a little olive oil.

# Summer Spaghetti with Tomato and Brie

PREPARATION about 20 minutes
COOKING about 15 minutes

300g/10oz spaghetti
500g/1lb 2oz courgettes
2 tbsp olive oil
2 garlic cloves, thinly sliced
finely grated zest and juice of 1 lemon
6 ripe tomatoes, roughly chopped
100g/4oz Brie, diced

1 Cook the spaghetti in boiling salted water for 10–12 minutes until tender but still firm to the bite.
2 Meanwhile, cut the courgettes in half lengthwise, then cut into slices. Heat the oil in a large frying pan, then fry the courgettes and garlic for 3–4 minutes until softened. Add the lemon zest, tomatoes and about 3 tablespoons of the pasta water (enough to make a sauce-like consistency). Cook for 2–3 minutes more until the tomatoes begin to soften.
3 Remove from the heat and stir in the Brie so it just starts to melt, then season to taste with salt, pepper and lemon juice.
4 Drain the spaghetti well and add to the tomato sauce mixture. Toss well together, divide between bowls and serve.

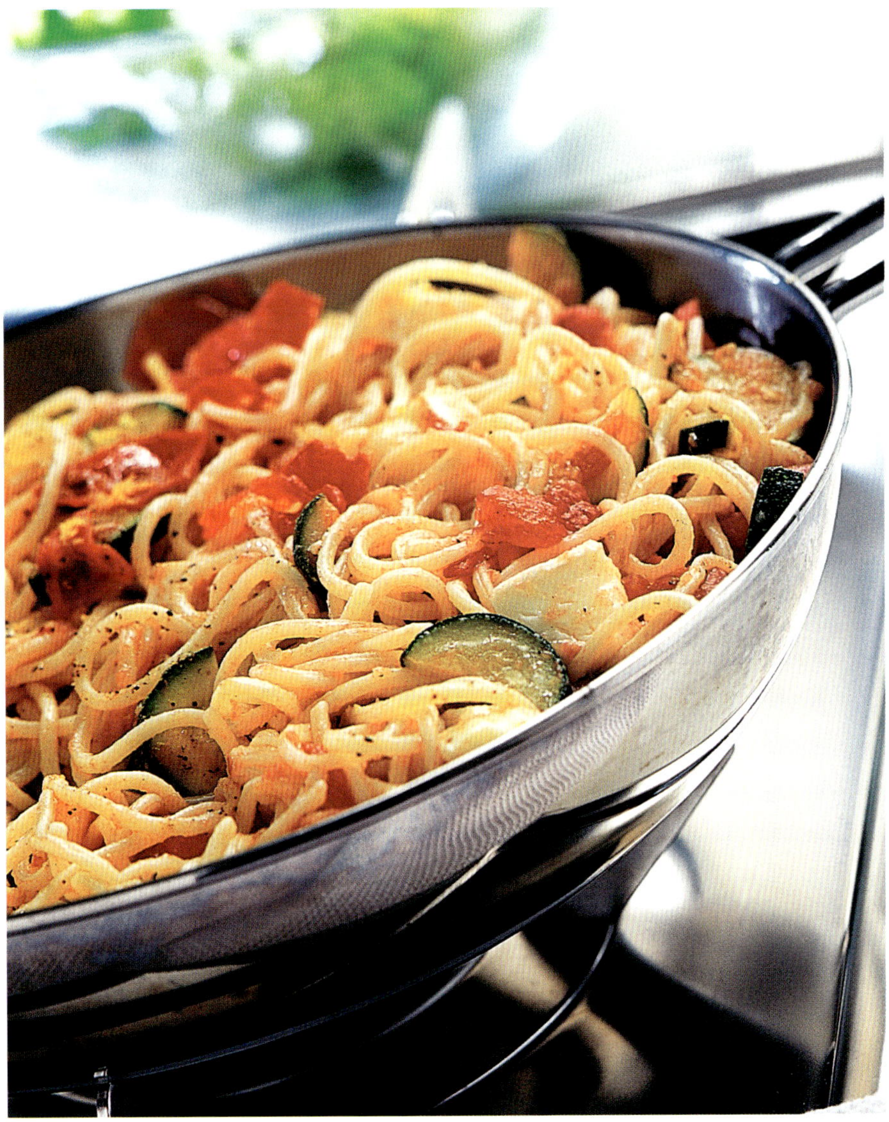

PER SERVING
**433 kcalories**
**protein 17g**
**carbohydrate 62g**
**fat 14g**
**saturated fat 5g**
**fibre 5g**
**added sugar none**
**salt 0.48g**

# Spicy Pepper Penne

**PER SERVING**
**546 kcalories**
**protein 21g**
**carbohydrate 79g**
**fat 19g**
**saturated fat 3g**
**fibre 7g**
**added sugar none**
**salt 1.32g**

**PREPARATION** 15 minutes
**COOKING** 25–30 minutes

**Chorizo gives a delightful spicy kick, but you could use the same quantity of thinly sliced salami if you prefer. Vegetarians, or those concerned about fat content, could replace the meat with anchovies, capers or olives.**

3 tbsp olive oil, plus more for greasing
3 red peppers, deseeded and cut into 1cm/½in-wide strips
1 large onion, thinly sliced
2 garlic cloves, crushed
two 400g/14oz cans of chopped tomatoes
300g/10oz penne or rigatoni
85g/3oz sliced chorizo
1 slice of white bread, made into crumbs
2 tbsp chopped fresh rosemary or 2 tsp dried
30g/1oz freshly grated Parmesan cheese

1 Preheat the oven to 200°C/400°F/Gas 6. Heat 2 tablespoons of the oil in a pan and cook the peppers and onion for 10 minutes until soft and golden, shaking the pan occasionally. Stir in the garlic and cook for 1 minute. Add the tomatoes and heat through. Season.
2 Meanwhile, cook the pasta according to the packet instructions until tender but still firm to the bite. Drain well and mix with the sauce and chorizo. Spoon into an oiled large shallow ovenproof dish.
3 Mix together the breadcrumbs, rosemary and Parmesan, then sprinkle over the pasta. Drizzle with the remaining oil and bake for 15–20 minutes until golden.

# Double Cheese and Tuna Pasta

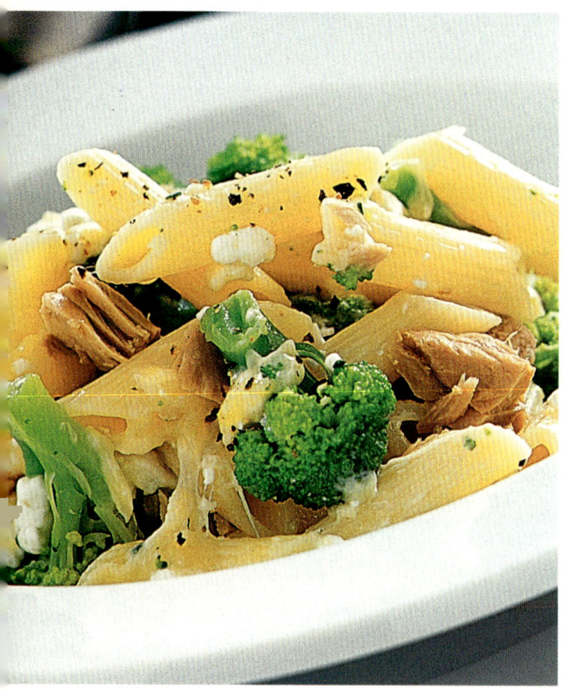

**PREPARATION** 5 minutes
**COOKING** 10–12 minutes

300g/10oz dried pasta quills (penne)
350g/12 oz broccoli florets
250g/9oz tub of low-fat cottage cheese with chives
100g/4oz mature Cheddar cheese, grated
200g/7 oz can of tuna in brine, drained

**VARIATIONS**
Try adding chopped stoned green or black olives or drained and rinsed capers to this dish just before serving.

1 Bring a large pan of salted water to the boil. Add the pasta, stir well, then boil for 10–12 minutes until just tender but still firm to the bite, adding the broccoli florets to the pan for the last 3–4 minutes of cooking.
2 Drain the pasta and broccoli then return them to the hot pan. Gently stir in the cottage cheese and Cheddar so they melt into the pasta. Carefully mix in the chunks of tuna, trying not to break them up too much. Season with salt and freshly ground black pepper.

**PER SERVING**
**482 kcalories • protein 37g • carbohydrate 61g**
**fat 12g • saturated fat 6g • fibre 5g**
**added sugar none • salt 1.51g**

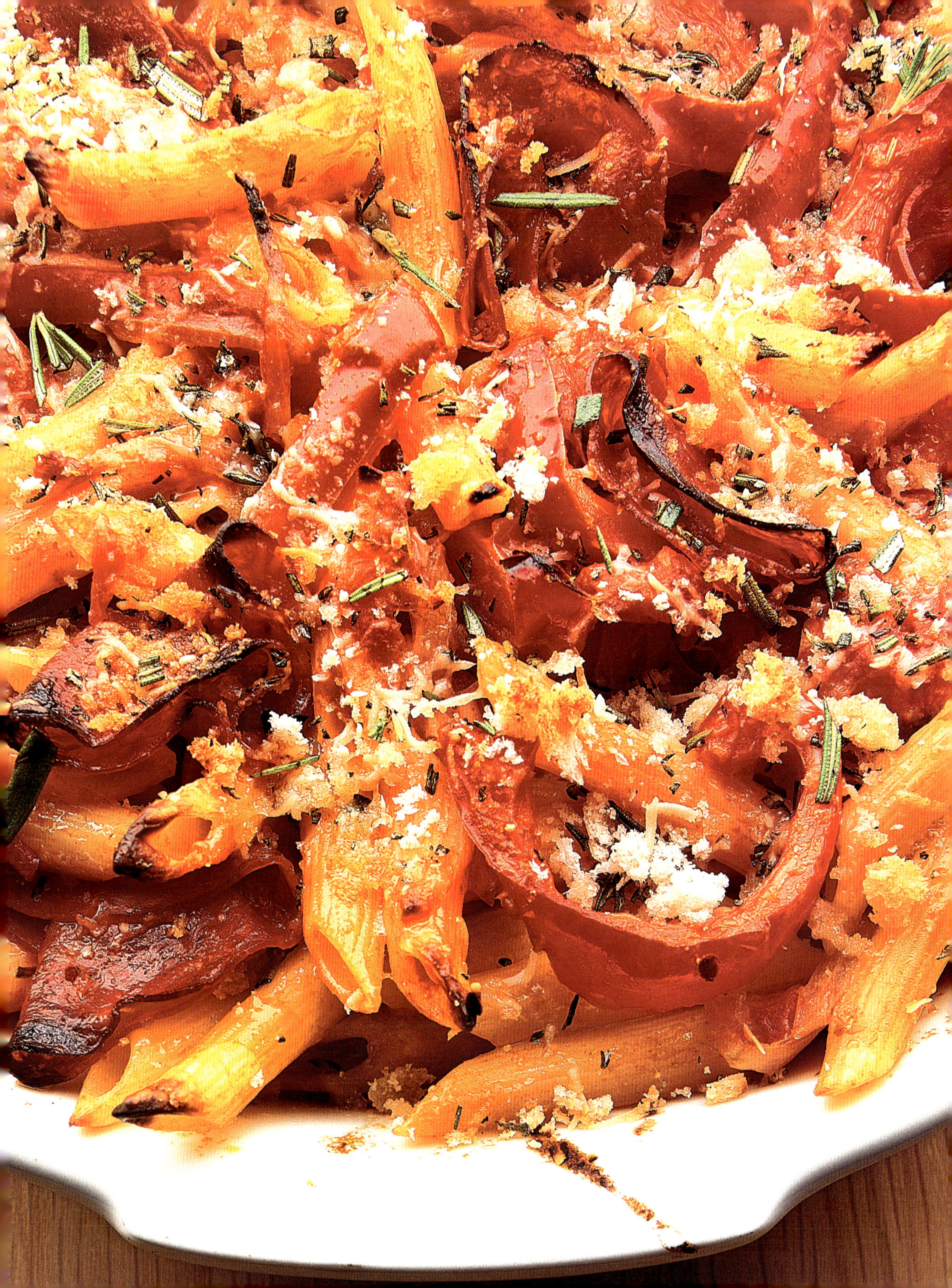

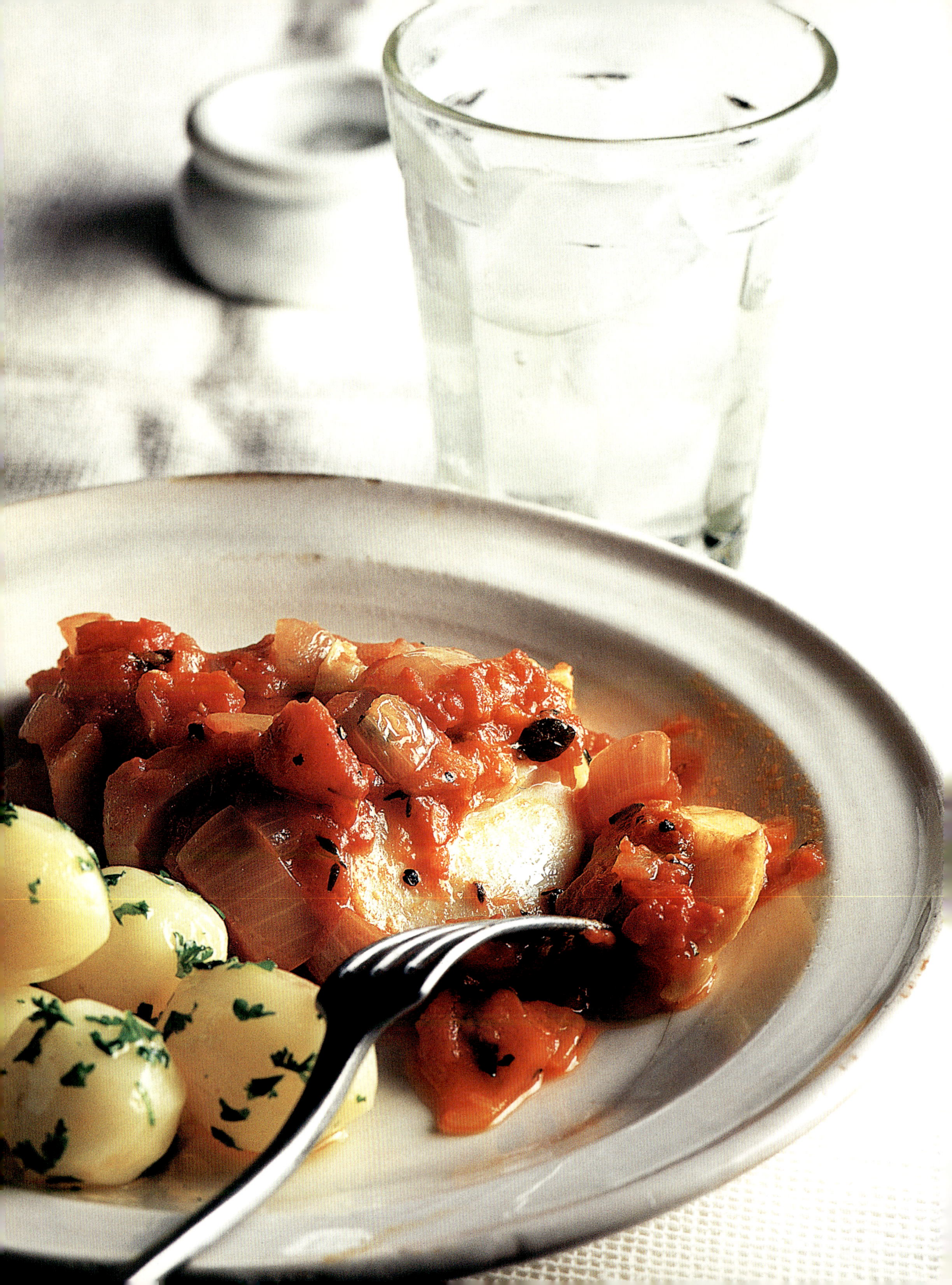

# Cod and Tomato Stew

PER SERVING
297 kcalories
protein 33g
carbohydrate 22g
fat 9g
saturated fat 1g
fibre 3g
added sugar none
salt 1.07g

**White fish is a good low-fat source of protein and is packed full of vitamins and minerals. The quality of the tomatoes makes a real difference in a dish this simple. Avoid the cheaper canned tomatoes as the juices are often watery and flavourless. If you find this is the case, add a little tomato purée to bump up the flavour. When fresh tomatoes come into season, you can use 450g/1lb instead of the canned variety – skin and chop them first.**

PREPARATION 5 minutes
COOKING about 25 minutes

2 tbsp olive oil
2 onions, chopped
400g/14oz can of chopped tomatoes
1 tbsp soy sauce
1 tsp fresh thyme, chopped, or 1/2 tsp dried
4 skinless cod fillets, each about 175g/6oz

1 Heat the oil in a wide pan, then fry the onions for 10 minutes, stirring occasionally, until they are well softened and lightly browned.
2 Stir in the tomatoes, soy sauce, thyme, salt and pepper. Bring to the boil, stir well, then simmer uncovered for 5 minutes until the mixture has thickened slightly.
3 Slide the cod fillets into the pan, cover with a lid or foil and cook gently for about 5 minutes, until the cod is tender and flakes easily.
4 Serve with floury potatoes or noodles.

# Trout with Warm Potato Salad

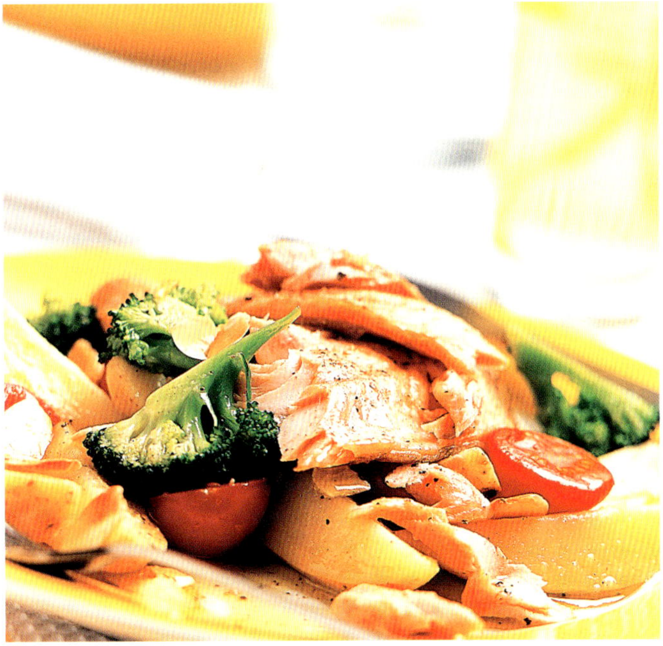

PREPARATION about 15 minutes
COOKING 12 minutes

575g/1 1/4lb new potatoes
225g/8oz broccoli, cut into small florets
4 trout fillets, each about 100g/4oz
3 tbsp olive oil, plus more for brushing
1 tbsp white wine vinegar
12 cherry tomatoes, halved
2 tbsp toasted flaked almonds

PER SERVING
378 kcalories
protein 26g
carbohydrate 26g
fat 19g
saturated fat 2g
fibre 4g
added sugar none
salt 0.43g

1 Cut the potatoes in half, or quarters if large. Cook in a pan of boiling salted water for 12 minutes, adding the broccoli for the last 3 minutes of cooking time.
2 Meanwhile, preheat the grill to high. Put the trout fillets on the grill pan. Brush each with a little oil and season with salt and black pepper. Grill for 3–4 minutes.
3 Drain the vegetables well. Tip into a bowl. Whisk together the oil and vinegar. Add to the hot vegetables with the tomatoes, almonds and a little seasoning. Toss well and serve with the grilled trout.

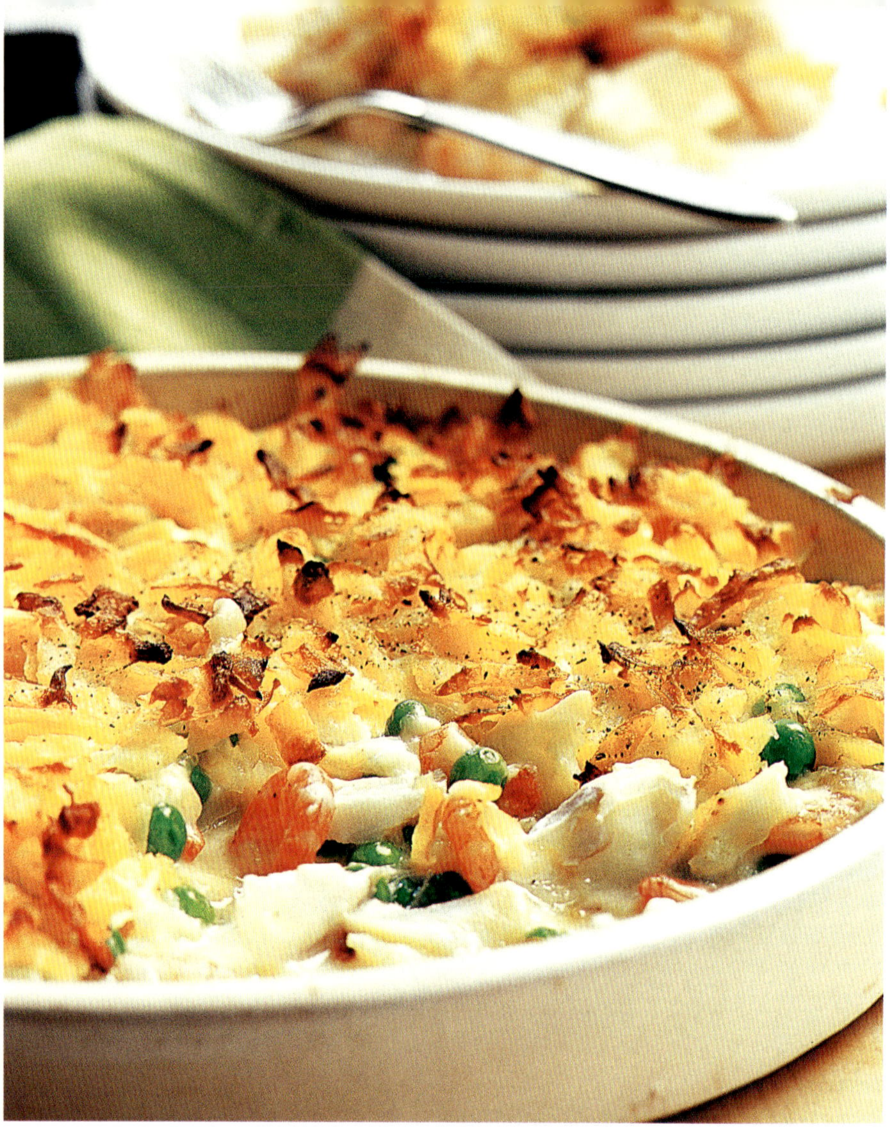

PER SERVING
533 kcalories
protein 49g
carbohydrate 51g
fat 16g
saturated fat 4g
fibre 5g
added sugar none
salt 3.74g

# Quick Fish Pie

**Easy comfort food, but with the fish, prawns and peas it has a wide range of nutrients – yet is relatively low in fat. Don't add salt as the smoked fish and potatoes have lots.**

SERVES 2
(easily doubled)
PREPARATION
10 minutes
COOKING
about 35 minutes

250g/9oz smoked haddock
250ml/9fl oz skimmed milk
100g/4oz large peeled cooked prawns
85g/3oz frozen peas
knob of butter
1 tbsp plain flour
4 tbsp low-fat natural fromage frais
400g/14oz pack of potato sauté

VARIATIONS

You could use haddock or cod fillets instead of the smoked haddock.

1 Preheat the oven to 200°C/400°F/Gas 6. Gently poach the haddock in the milk for 5 minutes. Remove with the slotted spoon, reserving the milk. Discarding the skin, flake the flesh into large chunks. Put these, the prawns and peas in the base of a heatproof dish.

2 Heat the butter in a small pan, then stir in the flour. Cook for 1 minute, stirring continuously, then gradually stir in the reserved milk. Bring to the boil, stirring to make a smooth thick sauce. Stir in the fromage frais, season to taste and pour over the fish.

3 Crumble the potatoes over the top of the fish, then bake for 25 minutes until bubbling and golden.

# Cod Fillets with Pan-fried Cabbage

PER SERVING
**241 kcalories**
**protein 31g**
**carbohydrate 4g**
**fat 11g**
**saturated fat 5g**
**fibre 3g**
**added sugar none**
**salt 1.1g**

PREPARATION about 10 minutes
COOKING 12–15 minutes

30g/1oz butter
4 rashers of streaky bacon, chopped
1 small Savoy cabbage, shredded
150ml/¼ pint vegetable stock
4 skinned cod fillets, each about 150g/5oz
boiled potatoes, to serve

1 Heat half the butter in a large frying pan. Add the bacon and cook until crisp. This will take 3–5 minutes. Stir in the cabbage. Pour over the stock and cook, stirring, for 3 minutes until the cabbage is almost tender. Transfer to a microwavable heatproof dish.

2 Lay the fish on top of the cabbage. Dot with the remaining butter and season. Cover with film and microwave on High for 5 minutes or until the fish is cooked (the flesh will start to turn opaque). Serve with boiled potatoes.

VARIATION

If you have no microwave cooker, preheat the grill and put the cod fillets on a grill pan lined with buttered foil. Grill for 5–8 minutes, turning once, depending on the thickness of the fillets, until cooked through. Meanwhile, cook the cabbage for a further 4–5 minutes until tender in the pan.

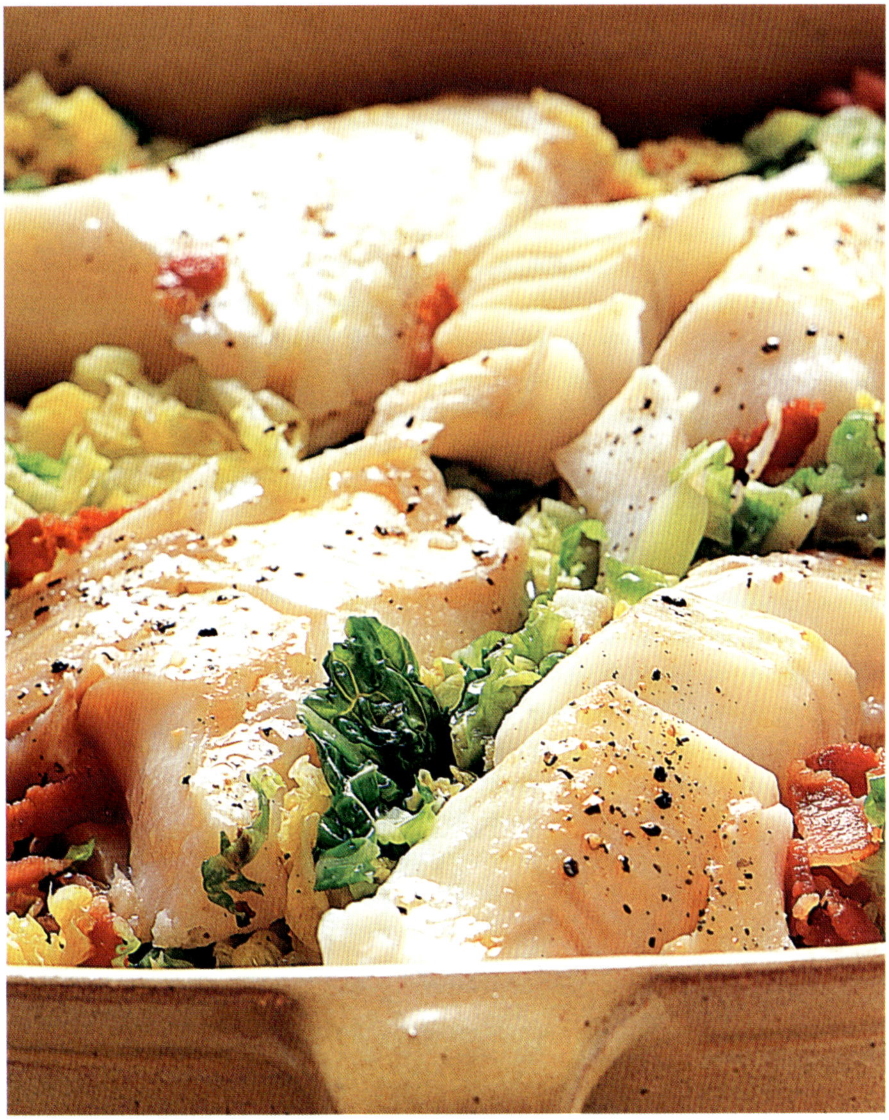

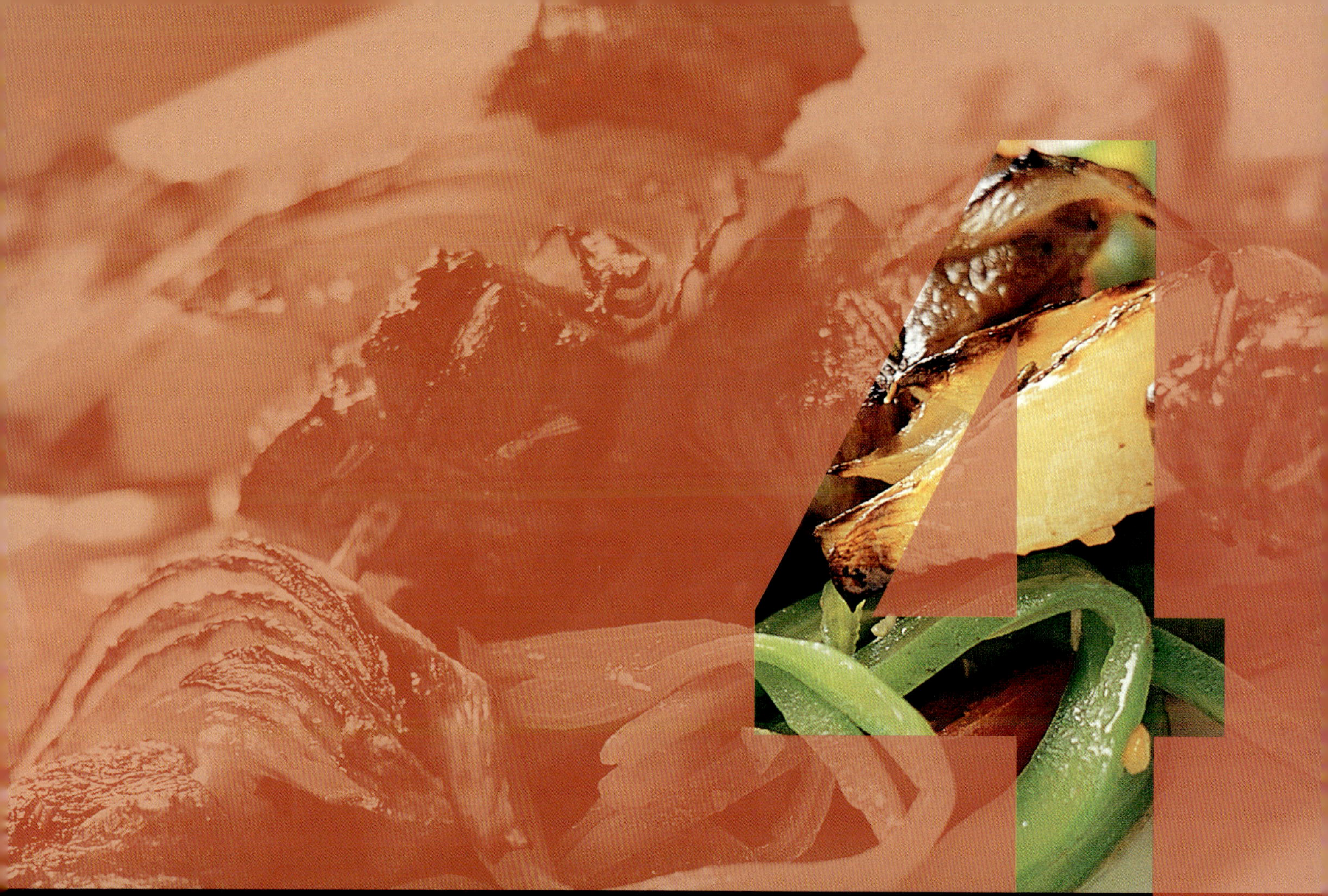

4

# Measured Midweek Specials and Sunday Lunches

*For meals that you need to be just that little bit special, like those marking a birthday or the big family gathering at the weekend, you will probably want to centre them around a traditional favourite like beef, lamb or pork. There are ways of making even these sinful saturated treats much better for you, so you can have the best of both worlds. One important answer lies in building in lots of good fresh vegetables and pulses, rather than just tagging on the sprouts cooked until they have no taste, no texture and no nutrients.*

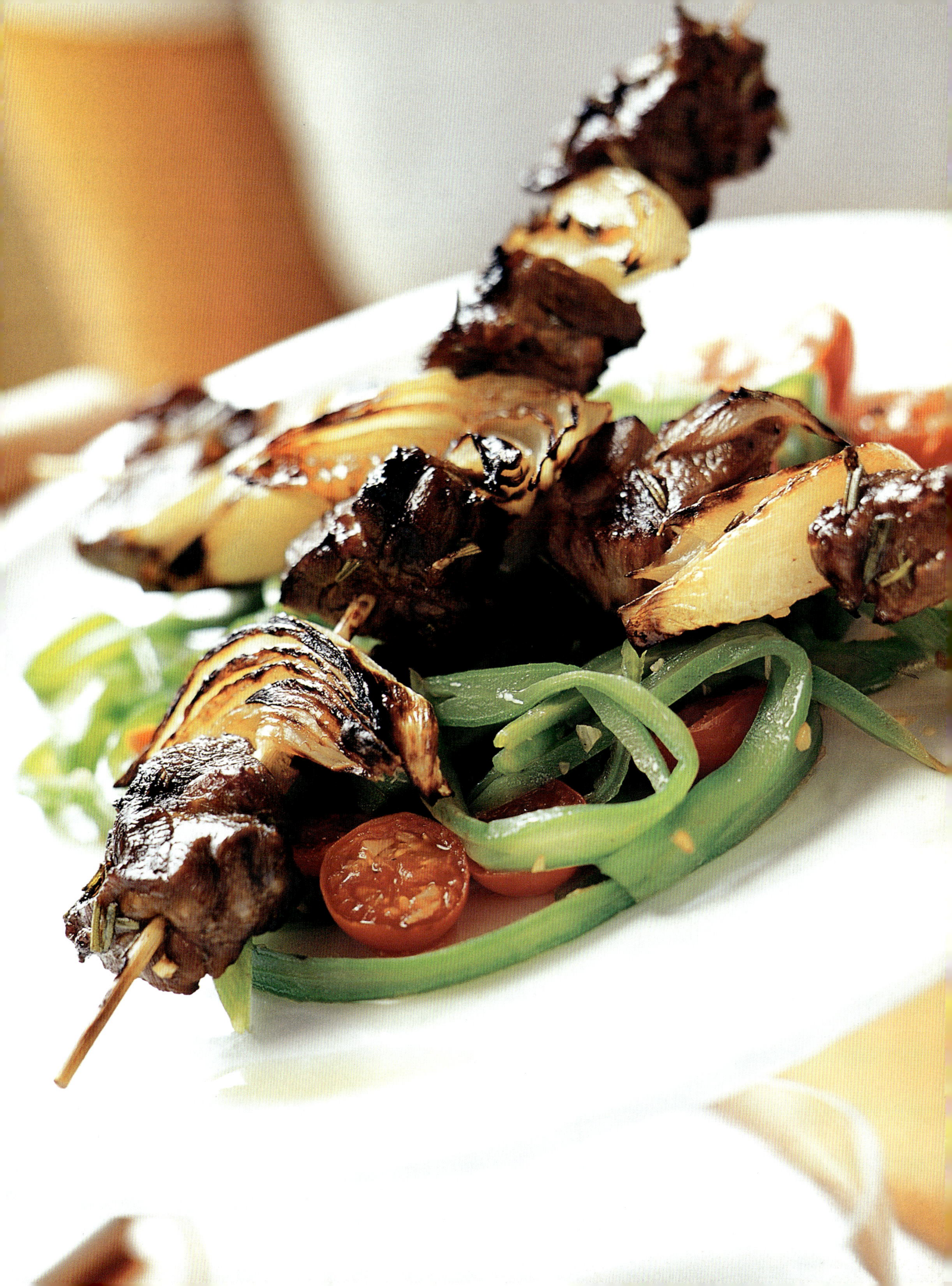

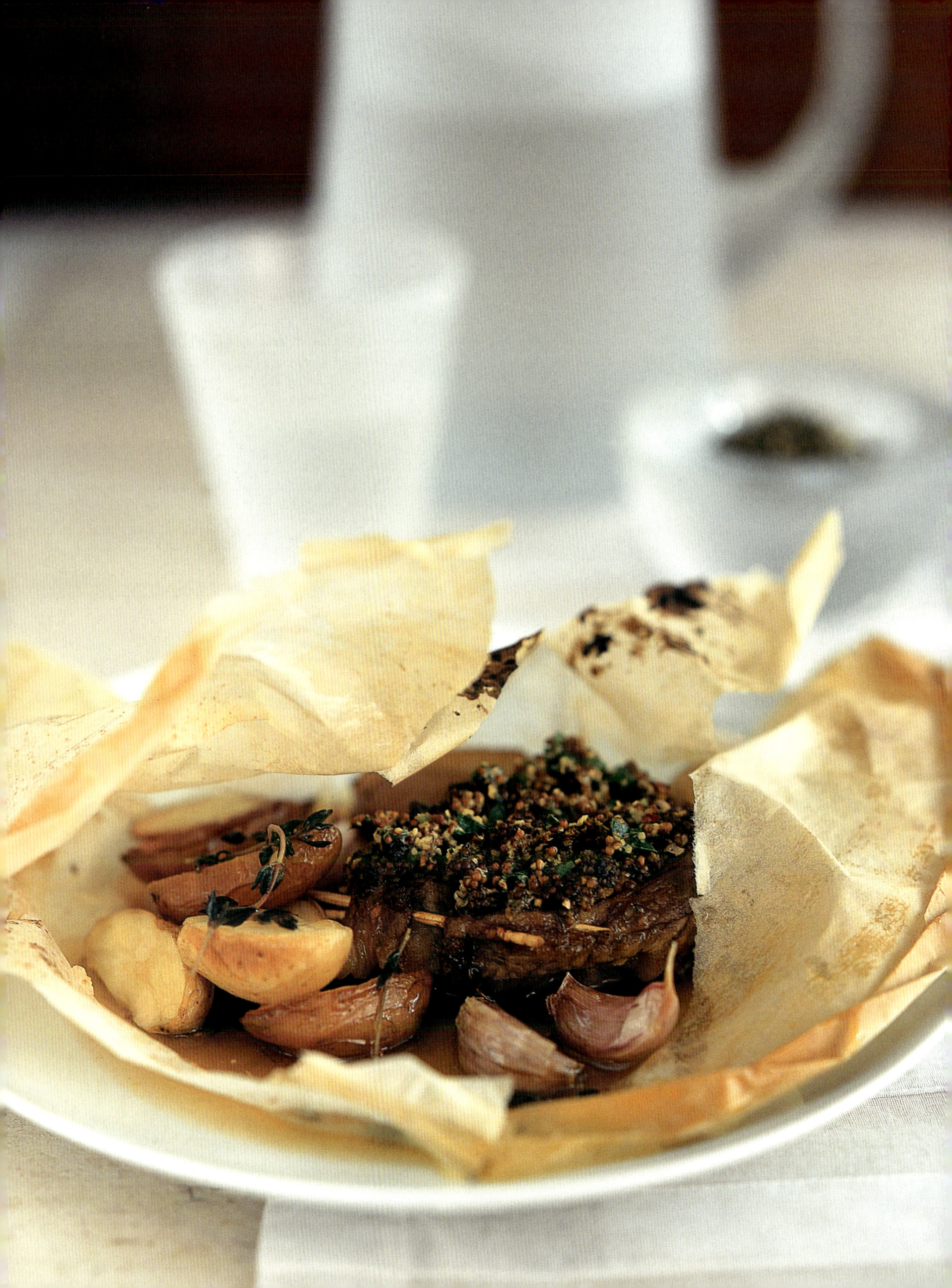

# Rosemary Lamb Kebabs with Runner Bean Spaghetti

PER SERVING
415 kcalories
protein 38g
carbohydrate 7g
fat 26g
saturated fat 9g
fibre 3g
added sugar none
salt 0.32g

**As lamb has such a high fat content, it is more often than not largely ignored in healthy-eating regimes. Some cuts of lamb are, however, significantly leaner than others - leg being about 30% leaner than shoulder, for instance. Fat content aside, lamb is a good source of the B vitamins, iron and zinc. It is also quite possibly a healthier bet among meats as it is one of the few that has more or less resisted intensive farming methods.**

PREPARATION about 25 minutes
COOKING 12–15 minutes

4 tbsp olive oil
3 sprigs of rosemary, chopped
1 tbsp balsamic vinegar
700g/1lb 9oz lean boneless lamb (leg or fillet), cubed
1 onion, cut into wedges
450g/1lb runner beans
100g/4oz cherry tomatoes
1 garlic clove, chopped
warm focaccia, to serve

1 Preheat the grill or barbecue to hot. Put half the oil in a large bowl with the rosemary, vinegar, salt and pepper. Whisk to mix, add the lamb and the onions and mix well.
2 Thread the lamb and onion wedges on 4–8 skewers. Grill or barbecue for 12–15 minutes, turning occasionally, until the lamb is tender and nicely browned.
3 While the kebabs are cooking, put the runner beans through a bean stringer or cut them into long thin strips. Halve the tomatoes. Cook the beans in a pan of boiling salted water for 5–6 minutes until just tender. Drain well.
4 Heat the remaining oil in a pan and fry the garlic briefly. Add the tomatoes and cook gently until just softened. Stir in the beans and season. Heat through and serve with the kebabs and warm focaccia.

# Mustard and Pepper Crusted Lamb with New Potatoes

PREPARATION 30 minutes
COOKING 30 minutes

4 lean lamb chump chops, each about 150g/5oz
2 tbsp olive oil
1 tbsp mixed peppercorns, crushed
4 tbsp wholegrain mustard
2 tbsp chopped fresh parsley
550g/1¼lb new potatoes
8–12 garlic cloves, in their skins
fresh thyme sprigs
coarse salt
green beans or broad beans, to serve

PER SERVING
371 kcalories • protein 29g • carbohydrate 27g
fat 17g • saturated fat 5g • fibre 3g
added sugar none • salt 1.25g

1 Preheat the oven to 190°C/375°F/Gas 5. Trim any excess fat from the chops. To give each chop a nice round shape, tuck the ends in and secure them with a small wooden cocktail stick.
2 Heat 1 tablespoon of the oil in a large frying pan. Add the chops and fry briefly over a high heat on each side just to seal and brown. Remove from the heat and set aside.
3 Mix the peppercorns with the mustard and parsley. Spread the mixture over the top of each lamb chop.
4 Cut out four 35cm/14in circles from sheets of baking parchment or greaseproof paper and brush one side of each circle lightly with oil. Slice the potatoes lengthwise - the slices should be the thickness of a £1 coin (if the potatoes are small just cut them in half). Toss with the garlic cloves in the remaining oil.
5 Divide the potatoes and garlic between each paper circle. Tuck in the thyme sprigs and sprinkle with coarse salt and black pepper. Sit the lamb chops to one side (don't put them on top or this will slow down the cooking of the potatoes), then fold the paper over to enclose everything, making sure the cocktail sticks don't pierce the paper. Twist the paper edges to seal completely.
6 Put the parcels on a baking sheet and bake for 30–40 minutes. Serve with green or broad beans.

# Spicy Beef with Pumpkin and Corn

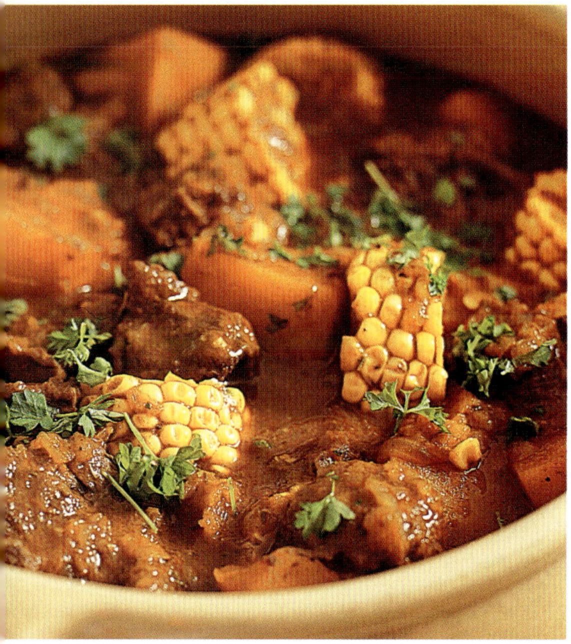

**This casserole is so mildly spiced it is unlikely to offend anyone, but for those who like extra heat, put the bottle of Tabasco, red or green (or both), on the table, so that they can pep up their serving.**

PER SERVING
**433 kcalories • protein 52g • carbohydrate 18g fat 18g • saturated fat 6g • fibre 3g added sugar none • salt 1.16g**

SERVES 6
PREPARATION 20 minutes
COOKING 2 hours 20 minutes

1.3kg/3lb braising beef
1 tbsp seasoned flour
2 tbsp olive oil
2 onions, sliced
2 garlic cloves, chopped
900ml/1½ pints beef or vegetable stock
2 tbsp tomato purée
1 tbsp paprika
2 tsp dried oregano
900g/2lb pumpkin
3 ears of corn on the cob
1 tsp Tabasco sauce, plus more for serving
chopped parsley, to serve

1 Cut the beef into 4cm/1½in chunks and toss in the seasoned flour. Heat the oil in a large pan which has a tight-fitting lid. Fry the beef, in batches if necessary, on all sides until well browned.
2 Add the onions and stir well. Cook for about 5 minutes, stirring in the garlic about halfway through.
3 Stir in the stock, tomato purée, paprika and oregano. Bring to the boil, then cover tightly and simmer for 1½ hours.
4 About halfway through the cooking time, peel and deseed the pumpkin. Cut the flesh into 4cm/1½in chunks, add to the casserole and return to the boil. Cook for a further 30 minutes.
5 Cut the corn across into 4cm/1½in slices and add to the casserole with the Tabasco. Cook for a further 10–15 minutes, then taste and adjust the seasoning and sprinkle with parsley.

# Oriental Stir-fried Lamb with Mushrooms

PER SERVING
**300 kcalories
protein 28g
carbohydrate 7g
fat 16g
saturated fat 6g
fibre 1g
added sugar none
salt 2.95g**

**Cutting the meat into thin slivers means it absorbs all the oriental flavours of the marinade in the time it takes you to prepare the rest of the meal.**

SERVES 6
PREPARATION 10 minutes, plus 20 minutes' marinating
COOKING 10 minutes

750g/1lb 10oz lean lamb steaks, cut into thin strips
6 tbsp dry sherry
6 tbsp dark soy sauce
4 tsp sesame oil
1 tbsp cornflour
1 tbsp sesame seeds
1 tbsp vegetable oil
4 garlic cloves, finely chopped
1cm/½in piece of fresh root ginger, grated
225g/8oz horse or chestnut mushrooms, halved
bunch of spring onions, thinly sliced
boiled rice, to serve

1 Mix together the lamb, sherry, soy, sesame oil and cornflour. Leave for 20 minutes.
2 Heat a wok, then dry-fry the sesame seeds until golden brown. Remove and set aside.
3 Drain the meat, reserving the marinade. Heat the vegetable oil in a wok, then stir-fry the lamb for 3 minutes until browned.
4 Add the garlic, ginger, mushrooms, half the spring onions and the marinade, and cook for 2 minutes until the onions start to soften.
5 Sprinkle with sesame seeds and the remaining spring onions. Serve with boiled rice.

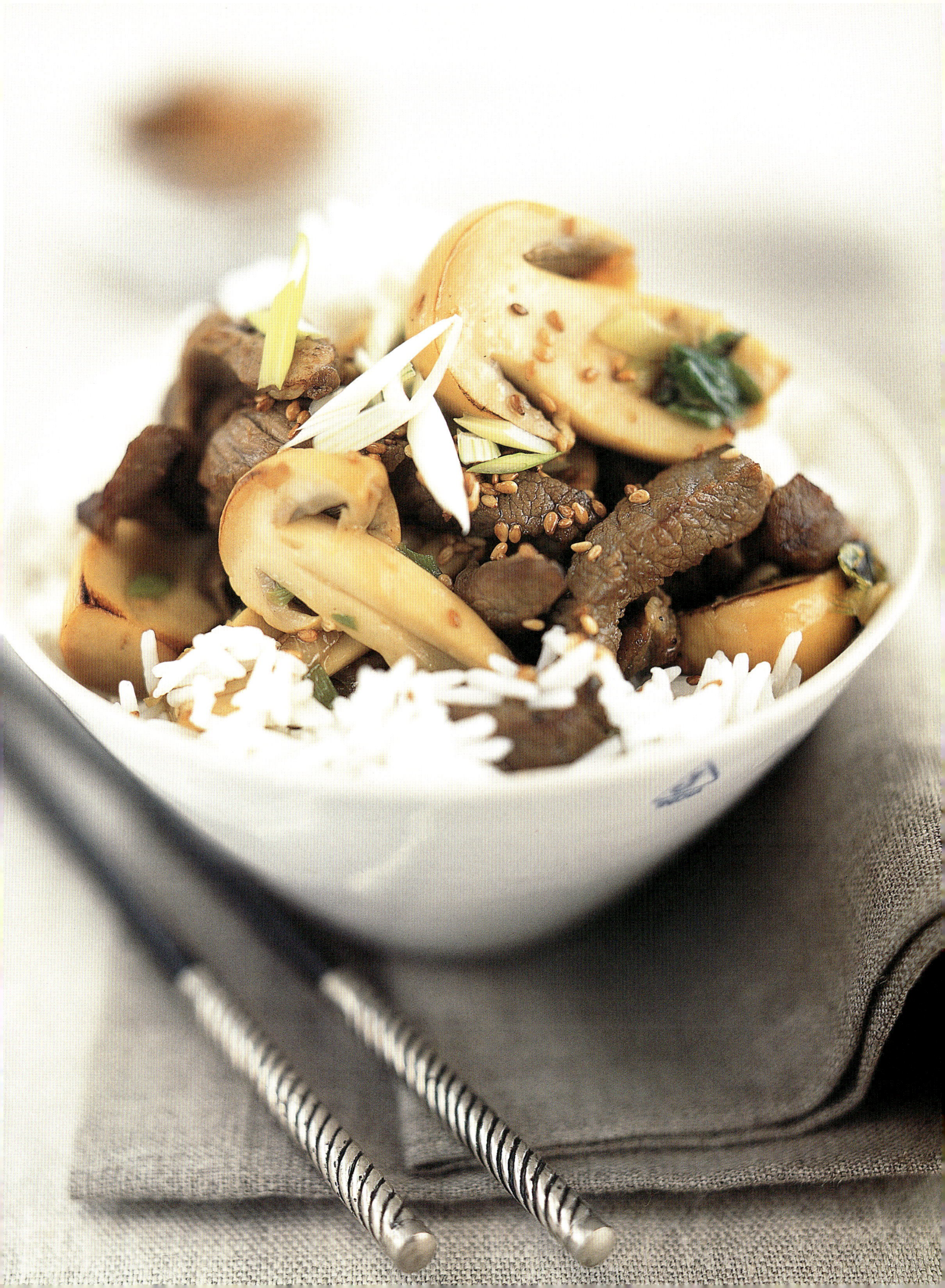

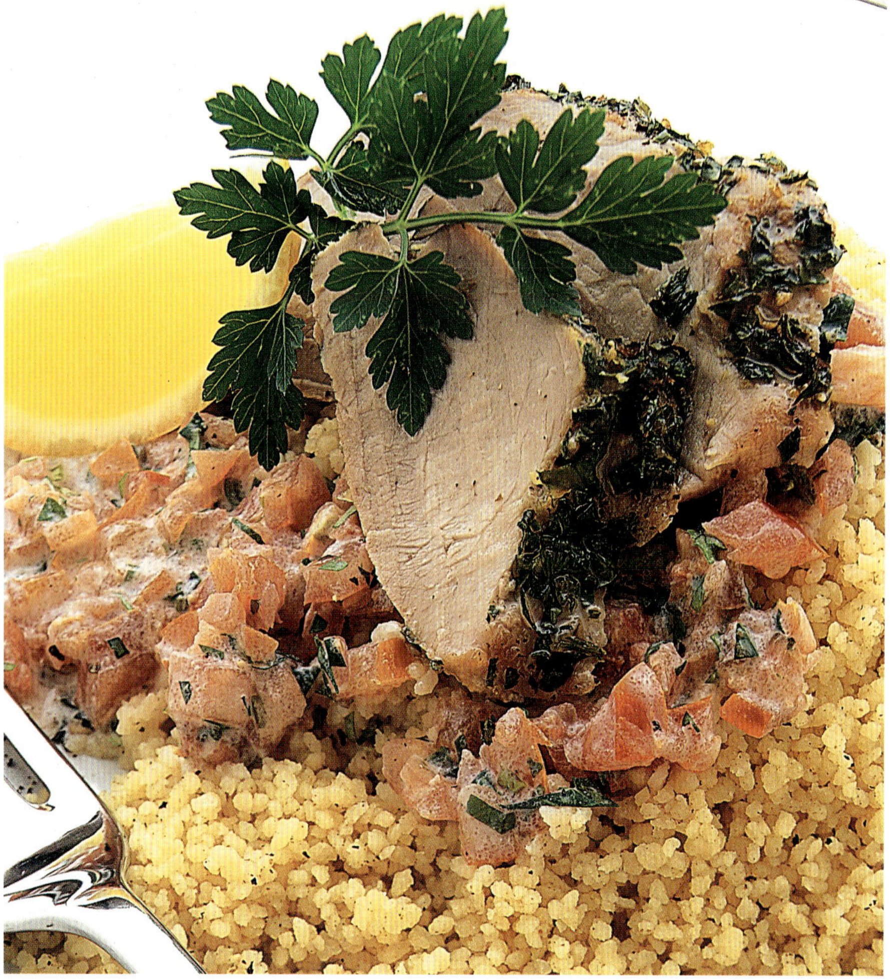

**PER SERVING**
**338 kcalories**
**protein 31g**
**carbohydrate 34g**
**fat 9g**
**saturated fat 2g**
**fibre 1g**
**added sugar none**
**salt 0.54g**

# Pork Tenderloin with Herb Crust and Tomato Dressing

**Today's pork fillet is lower in fat than beef, and a good source of B vitamins and zinc.**

PREPARATION 30 minutes
COOKING 25 minutes

2 tsp olive oil, plus 1 tbsp to serve
1 large pork tenderloin, about 450g/1lb, trimmed of fat and any membrane
zest of 1 lemon
5 tbsp chopped fresh flat-leaf parsley, plus a few sprigs to garnish
4 ripe plum tomatoes, finely chopped
4 tbsp natural low-fat yoghurt
1 tbsp finely chopped coriander
lemon juice and Tabasco sauce, to taste
½ tsp ground coriander
½ tsp ground cumin
300ml/½ pint chicken stock
225g/8oz couscous
lemon wedges, to serve

1 Preheat the oven to 200°C/400°F/Gas 6. Rub the 2 teaspoons of oil over the pork; season. Mix together the lemon zest and 4 tablespoons of parsley and press firmly over the sides and top of the pork to coat generously. Cook in a roasting tin for about 25 minutes until done.
2 Make the dressing: mix together the tomatoes, yoghurt, coriander and remaining parsley. Season and add lemon juice and Tabasco to taste. Set aside.
3 While the pork is cooking, dry-fry the coriander and cumin in a pan over a low heat for about 2 minutes until aromatic. Add the stock and bring to the boil with ½ teaspoon of salt. Put the couscous in a bowl and add the stock, then leave for 15 minutes. Stir with a fork, then add lemon juice to taste. Season and keep warm.
4 When the pork is done, leave it to rest for 2–3 minutes, then carve it at an angle into 8 slices.
5 Pile couscous on plates and drizzle with oil. Spoon over some tomato dressing (serve rest separately), lay pork on top and garnish with parsley. Serve with lemon wedges.

# Turkey and Sweet Potato Gratin

PREPARATION about 20 minutes
COOKING 25–30 minutes

900g/2lb sweet potatoes, peeled and chopped
550g/1 1/4lb Brussels sprouts, halved or quartered (depending on size)
1 tbsp olive oil
1 onion, sliced
225g/8oz cooked turkey, cut into chunks
25g/3/4oz butter, plus more for greasing
85g/3oz Stilton cheese

1 Cook the sweet potatoes in a pan of boiling salted water for 10–15 minutes. Add the sprouts and cook for 5 minutes more, until the vegetables are just tender.
2 Heat the oil in a frying pan and fry the onion for 4–5 minutes until golden. Stir in the turkey and heat through. Keep warm.
3 Preheat the grill and grease a shallow ovenproof dish with a little butter. Drain the vegetables, then mash roughly. Stir in the butter and season.
4 Spoon the vegetable mash into the prepared dish. Scatter the onion and turkey on top, then crumble over the Stilton and grill until the cheese has melted.

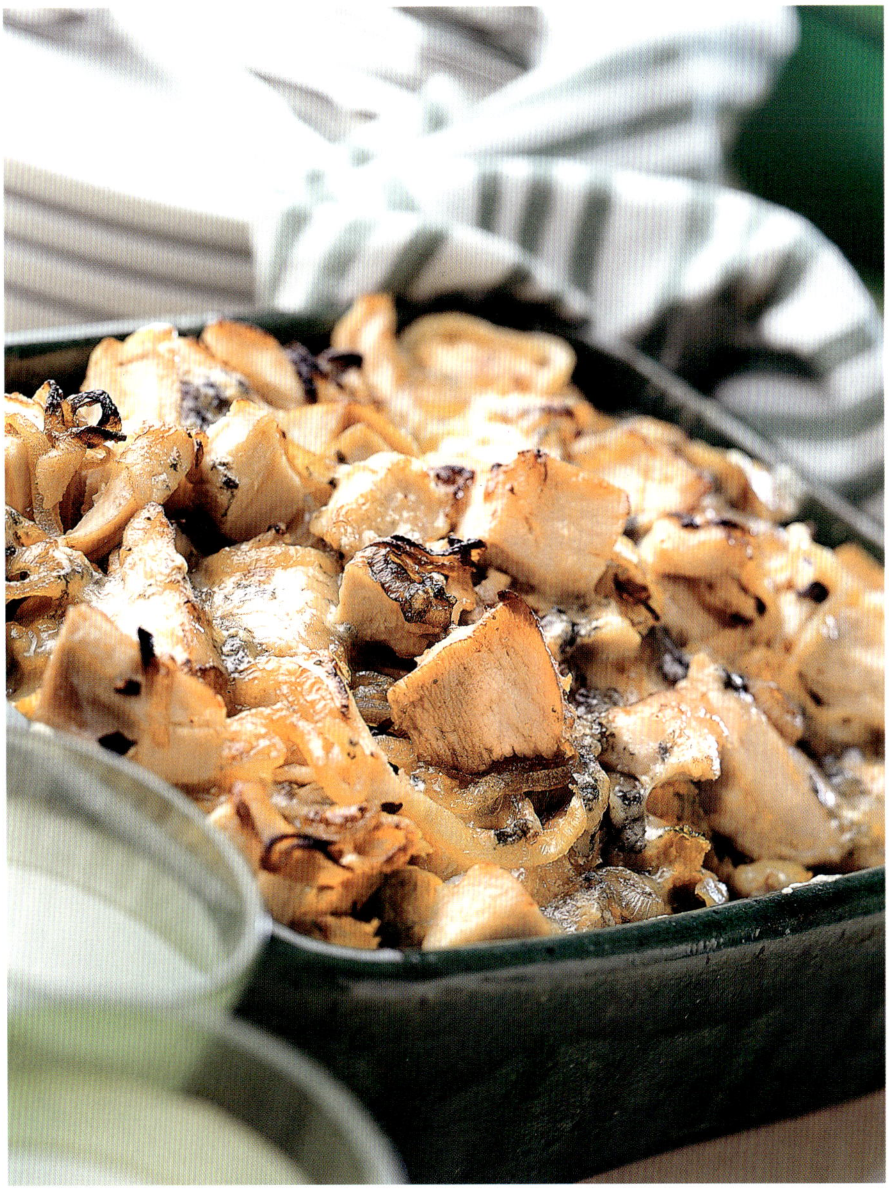

PER SERVING
**518 kcalories**
**protein 32g**
**carbohydrate 56g**
**fat 20g**
**saturated fat 10g**
**fibre 11g**
**added sugar none**
**salt 0.97g**

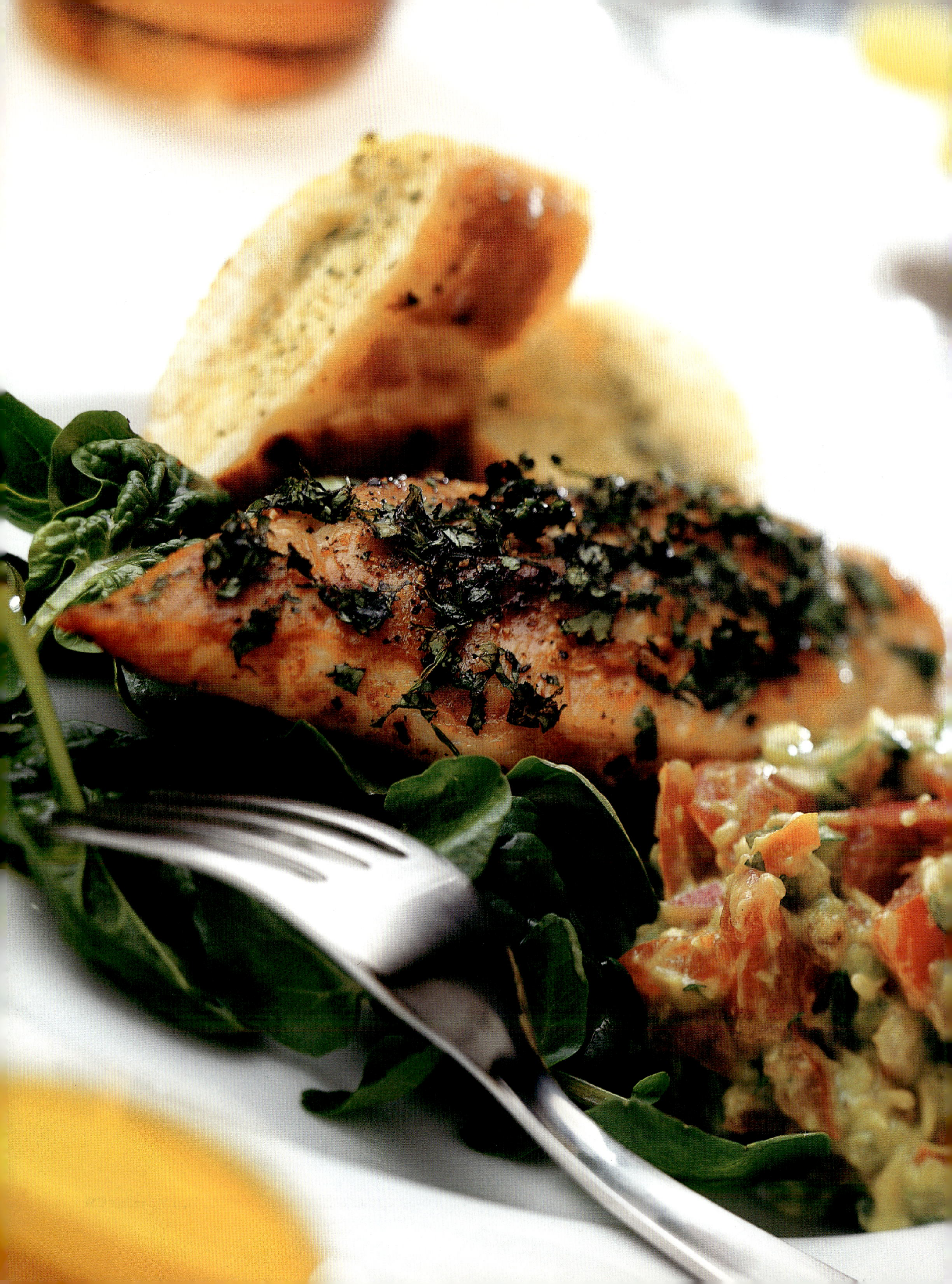

# Barbecued Coriander Chicken with Guacamole Salsa

PER SERVING
311 kcalories
protein 36g
carbohydrate 4g
fat 17g
saturated fat 2g
fibre 3g
added sugar none
salt 0.24g

PREPARATION
about 15 minutes

COOKING
20 minutes

**The raw vegetables in the salsa make this a very healthy dish. Avocado is a 'superfood' (see page 100), packed full of antioxidant vitamin E and monounsaturated fats.**

4 skinless chicken breast fillets, each about 150g/5oz
2 tbsp olive oil
2 tbsp finely chopped fresh coriander
125g/4½ oz mixed salad leaves
garlic bread, to serve

**for the guacamole salsa**

¼ red onion, roughly chopped
1 garlic clove, quartered
½–1 green chilli, deseeded
2 tomatoes, halved and deseeded
1 large, or 2 small, ripe avocados, peeled, stoned and roughly chopped
good handful of fresh coriander
2 tbsp fresh lemon juice

1 First cook the chicken: preheat the grill or barbecue. Brush the chicken with 1 tablespoon of the olive oil. Season well, then grill or barbecue for 20 minutes, turning halfway through. Sprinkle the coriander over the chicken for the last 5 minutes of cooking.
2 Make the salsa: put the onion, garlic and chilli in a food processor and pulse for a few seconds at a time to finely chop. Add the tomatoes, avocado, coriander and 1 tablespoon of lemon juice, and pulse until the ingredients are combined, but the mixture still has a chunky texture.
3 Empty the salad leaves into a bowl. Sprinkle over the remaining oil and lemon juice. Season well with salt and pepper. Toss well, then divide the salad between plates and serve with the chicken, guacamole salsa and garlic bread.

# Chinese Chicken Stir-fry

PER SERVING (FOR 4)
273 kcalories
protein 40g
carbohydrate 11g
fat 8g
saturated fat 4g
fibre 4g
added sugar none
salt 2.4g

SERVES 4–6 (easily halved)
PREPARATION about 15 minutes
COOKING about 10 minutes

30g/1oz butter (or 2 tbsp groundnut oil)
450g/1lb skinless chicken breast fillets, cut into thin strips
3 tbsp dark soy sauce
350g/12oz broccoli, broken into small florets
200g/7oz green beans, halved
1 bunch of spring onions, cut into long slices
2 tsp cornflour
juice of 2 oranges
30g/1oz fresh basil, roughly torn

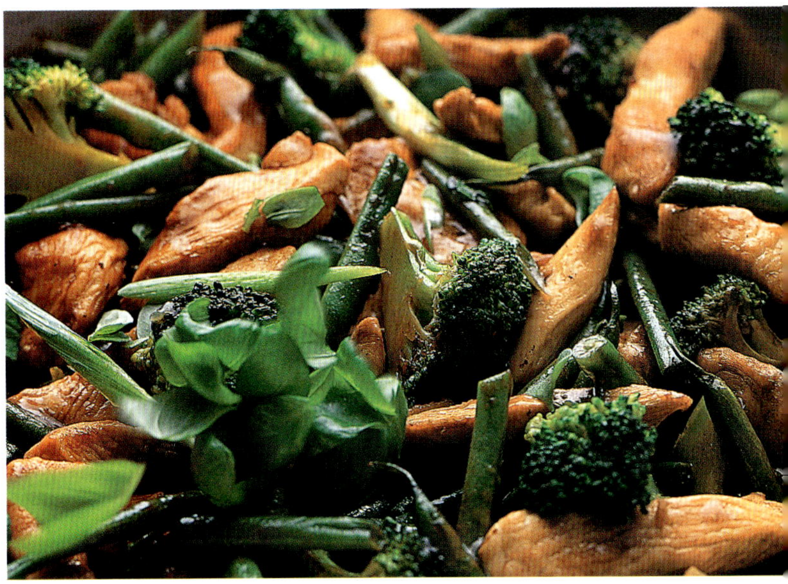

1 Heat the butter in a wok or large frying pan. Add the chicken strips and a splash of soy sauce and cook for 5 minutes, stirring, until the chicken starts to brown.
2 Stir in the broccoli, beans and half the spring onions and stir-fry for 3 minutes until just cooked.
3 Mix the cornflour with the orange juice and remaining soy sauce. Pour into the pan and continue to stir-fry for about 1 minute, until just thickened.
4 Scatter in the basil and remaining spring onions just before serving.

# Hot Toddy Chicken Breasts

PREPARATION 15–20 minutes
COOKING about 10 minutes

2 skinless chicken breast fillets
30g/1oz plain flour
grated zest and juice of 1 large lemon
15g/½oz butter
2 tbsp olive oil
100ml/3½fl oz whisky
2 heaped tsp clear honey
125ml/4fl oz good-quality chicken stock

**for the sautéed radicchio**

2 heads of radicchio
1 tbsp vegetable oil
85g/3oz streaky bacon, cut into strips

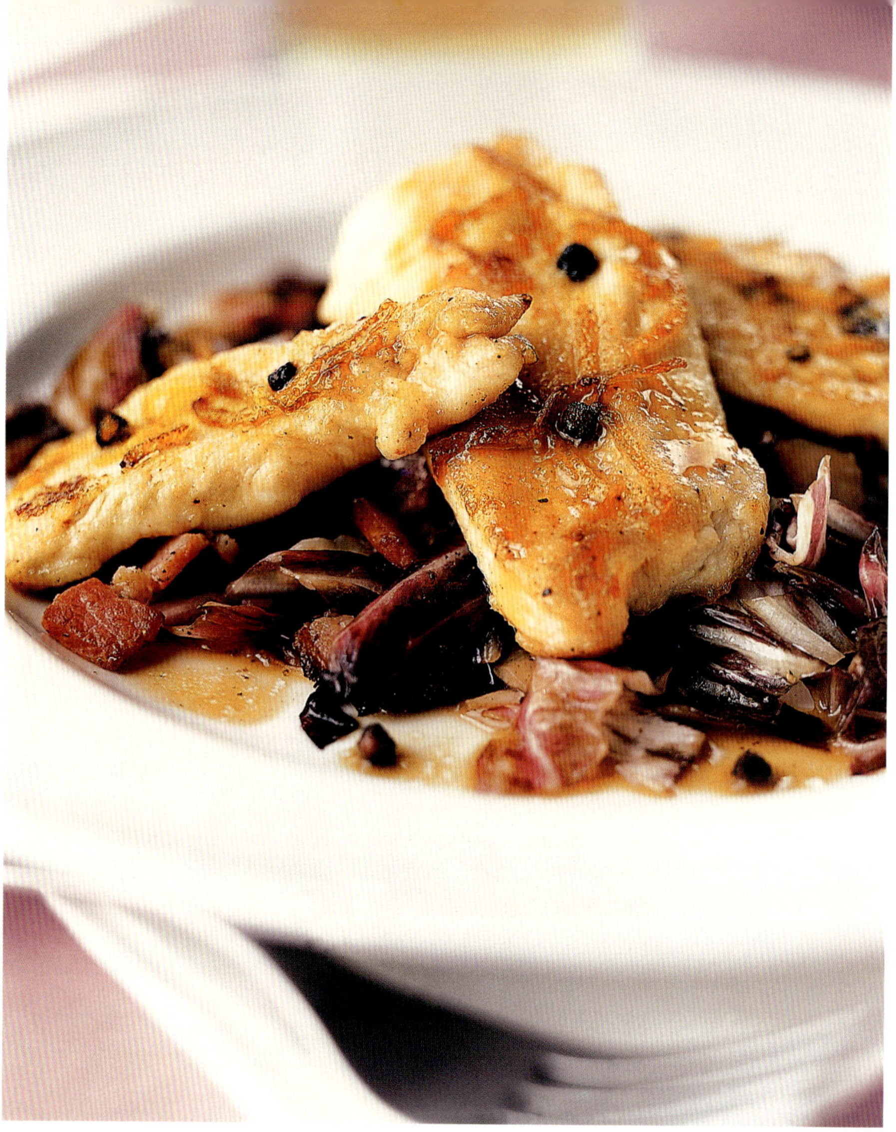

PER SERVING
**344 kcalories**
**protein 22g**
**carbohydrate 10g**
**fat 17g**
**saturated fat 5g**
**fibre 1g**
**added sugar 3g**
**salt 0.97g**

**When you add the whisky to this pan of chicken breasts, it makes a fine blaze. The whisky flavour lingers in the pan juices, making a tasty sauce with lemon and honey – the classic trio in a restorative hot toddy. Instead of the radicchio, try other bitter leaves, such as chicory, escarole or curly endive.**

1 Place the chicken fillets on a board and cut each at an angle into 3 slices. Put the slices between 2 sheets of plastic film and pound with a rolling pin to a thickness of about 3–5mm/⅛–¼in. On a plate, mix the flour with the lemon zest, salt and pepper. Toss the chicken in this and pat to discard the excess.

2 Heat half the butter and oil in a frying pan. Sauté half the chicken for about 1–2 minutes until golden. Turn and brown the other side. Transfer the chicken to a plate. Melt the remaining butter and oil, and fry the rest of the chicken.

3 Return all the chicken to the pan, then add the whisky and heat for ½–1 minute. Carefully set alight, then keep cooking until the flames die down. Transfer the chicken to a serving dish and keep warm.

4 Cook the radicchio: shred the heads, discarding the white core. Heat the oil in a frying pan and fry the bacon until it starts to brown. Add the radicchio and some black pepper and cook, stirring, for 1–2 minutes until the radicchio wilts slightly but is still a bit crisp. Taste and season, then cover with foil and keep warm.

5 Stir the lemon juice and honey into the chicken pan with the stock. Simmer until slightly thickened, stirring to dissolve the juices. Season to taste. Serve the chicken with the sauce and radicchio.

# Chicken, Fennel and Tomato Ragout

PREPARATION
20 minutes
COOKING
40 minutes

**This combination of flavours comes straight from the Mediterranean. The plain stew of chicken, fennel and tomato is excellent as it is, but for an extra burst of flavour sprinkle over a health-packed gremolata of lemon zest, chopped mint and garlic. Spoon it over polenta or mashed potatoes, with freshly grated Parmesan.**

4 chicken breast fillets, cut into large chunks
2 tbsp extra-virgin olive oil
1 onion, chopped
3 garlic cloves, finely chopped
1 tbsp coriander seeds, toasted and crushed
400g/14oz can of chopped tomatoes
1 tbsp tomato purée
$^{1}/_{2}$ tsp caster sugar
1 tbsp freshly chopped parsley
1 sprig of thyme
2 heads of fennel, trimmed and quartered
225g/8oz pitted black olives

**for the mint gremolata (optional)**
handful of mint, finely chopped
finely grated zest of 1 lemon
1 garlic clove, finely chopped

1 Brown the chicken pieces in the oil in a large pan. Transfer to a plate and set aside.
2 Reduce the heat and add the onion. Fry until almost tender, then add the garlic and coriander seeds. Fry for a further minute or so, then add 150ml/$^{1}/_{4}$ pint water, the tomatoes, tomato purée, sugar, parsley, thyme, salt and pepper.
3 Bring to the boil, add the chicken and the fennel, cover and simmer for 25 minutes or until both are cooked. Discard the thyme and add the olives. Season to taste.
4 Make the gremolata, if using it, by mixing together the ingredients. Sprinkle over the dish just before serving.

PER SERVING
**252 kcalories**
**protein 37g**
**carbohydrate 9g**
**fat 8g**
**saturated fat 1g**
**fibre 3g**
**added sugar 1g**
**salt 0.48g**

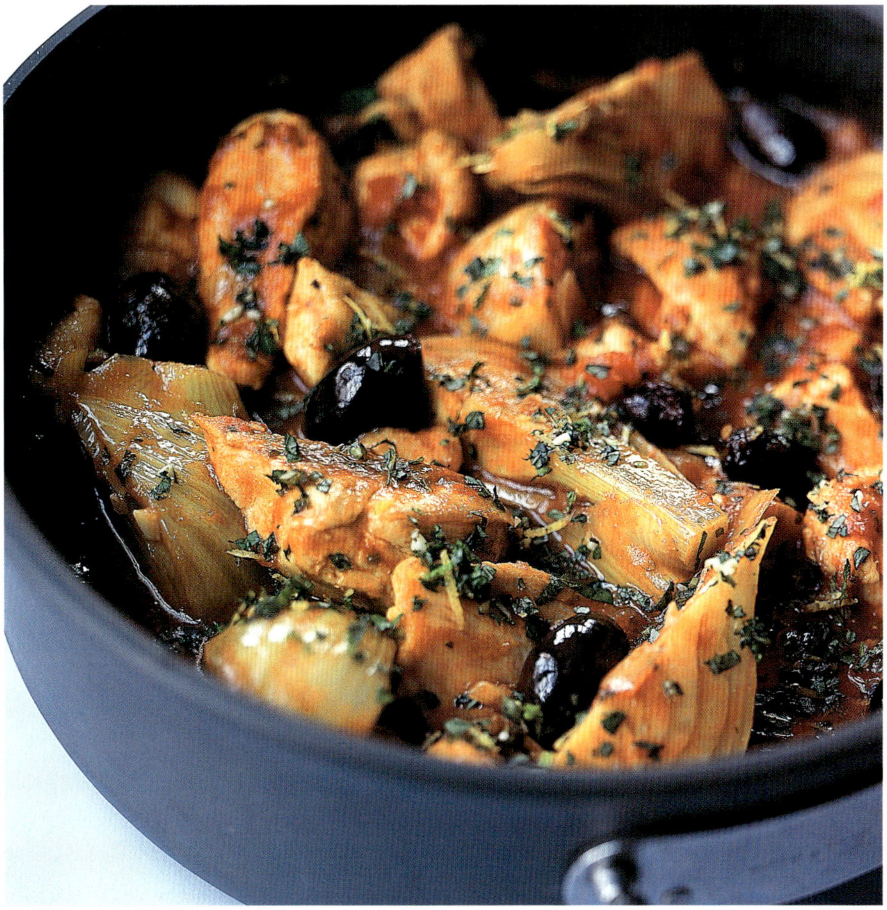

# Chicken with 40 Cloves of Garlic

PER SERVING
302 kcalories
protein 40g
carbohydrate 11g
fat 10g
saturated fat 4g
fibre 2g
added sugar 1g
salt 0.4g

**This sounds like an awful lot of garlic, but you'll be amazed at how deliciously sweet and mellow it tastes. The medicinal powers of garlic have been acknowledged for centuries, and today it is seen as one of our most valuable 'superfoods' (see page 100). Antibacterial, antiviral and antifungal, it also contains compounds that help lower blood cholesterol.**

PREPARATION 30 minutes
COOKING 1¼ hours

3 heads of garlic (to give about 40 cloves)
15g/½oz butter, plus an extra knob
1 tsp sugar
1 tbsp olive oil
4 chicken breast fillets
1 onion, finely chopped
100ml/3½fl oz chicken stock
100ml/3½fl oz white wine
2 sprigs of fresh thyme or a pinch of dried thyme
1 tbsp plain flour
good handful of chopped fresh parsley
boiled new potatoes, to serve

1 Preheat the oven to 160°C/325°F/Gas 3. Break the garlic into cloves, but don't peel them, and cook in a pan of boiling water for 3 minutes. Drain and peel. Set one aside and put the rest in an ovenproof dish with the knob of butter and the sugar. Bake at the bottom of the oven for 1¼ hours, shaking occasionally, until the garlic turns golden.
2 Meanwhile, prepare the chicken: heat the remaining butter and the oil in a casserole (which has a lid) big enough to hold all the breasts. Fry 2 chicken breasts, skin-side down, for 3–4 minutes, then turn and fry for 2–3 minutes more, spreading the breasts towards the end of frying to ensure they're evenly browned. Set aside and repeat with the remaining chicken. Remove from the dish.
3 Chop the reserved garlic clove. Cook the onion, covered, in the casserole for 5 minutes. Return the chicken to the dish with the stock, wine, thyme and garlic. Bring to a simmer, cover and put in the oven for about 35–40 minutes.
4 Transfer chicken to a dish. Boil the pan juices to reduce to about 300ml/½ pint. Remove the whole garlic cloves from their dish. Stir the flour into the garlic juices to make a paste, then add to the chicken juices, whisking until smooth and thick. Scatter chicken with garlic and coat with sauce. Sprinkle with parsley and serve with potatoes.

# Moroccan Chicken and Chickpeas

PER SERVING
539 kcalories
protein 39g
carbohydrate 52g
fat 21g
saturated fat 4g
fibre 6g
added sugar 3g
salt 1.12g

PREPARATION about 15 minutes
COOKING about 40 minutes

4 boneless skinless chicken thighs, 500g/1lb 2oz total weight
300ml/½ pint chicken or vegetable stock
2 onions, finely chopped
3 tbsp olive oil
1 tbsp clear honey
1 tsp each ground cumin and cinnamon
200g/7oz courgettes, cut into sticks
400g/14oz can of chickpeas, drained
3 tbsp chopped fresh parsley
juice of 1 lemon
cooked rice or couscous, to serve

1 Put the chicken, stock, onions, oil, honey and spices in a pan, and season. Bring to the boil, cover and cook gently for 25 minutes until the chicken is tender.
2 Add the courgettes and chickpeas and cook for 10 minutes.
3 Stir in the parsley and the lemon juice. Serve with rice or couscous.

# Chicken with a Red Pepper and Parsley Crust

PER SERVING
**210 kcalories**
**protein 23g**
**carbohydrate 5g**
**fat 11g**
**saturated fat 2g**
**fibre 1g**
**added sugar none**
**salt 0.19g**

PREPARATION about 10 minutes
COOKING 25 minutes

4 skinless chicken breast fillets
1 small red pepper, deseeded and roughly chopped
2 garlic cloves, finely chopped
large handful of fresh parsley
2 tbsp olive oil
pasta or new potatoes and a green salad, to serve

1 Preheat the oven to 200°C/400°F/Gas 6. Put the chicken breasts in a roasting tin or shallow ovenproof dish and season to taste with salt and pepper.
2 Put the red pepper, garlic and parsley in a food processor and pulse a few times until coarsely chopped. Stir in the oil and season generously with salt and pepper. Spread the crust over the chicken.
3 Spoon 2 tablespoons of water into the base of the dish and roast the chicken, uncovered, for 25 minutes.
4 Serve with pasta or new potatoes and a green salad.

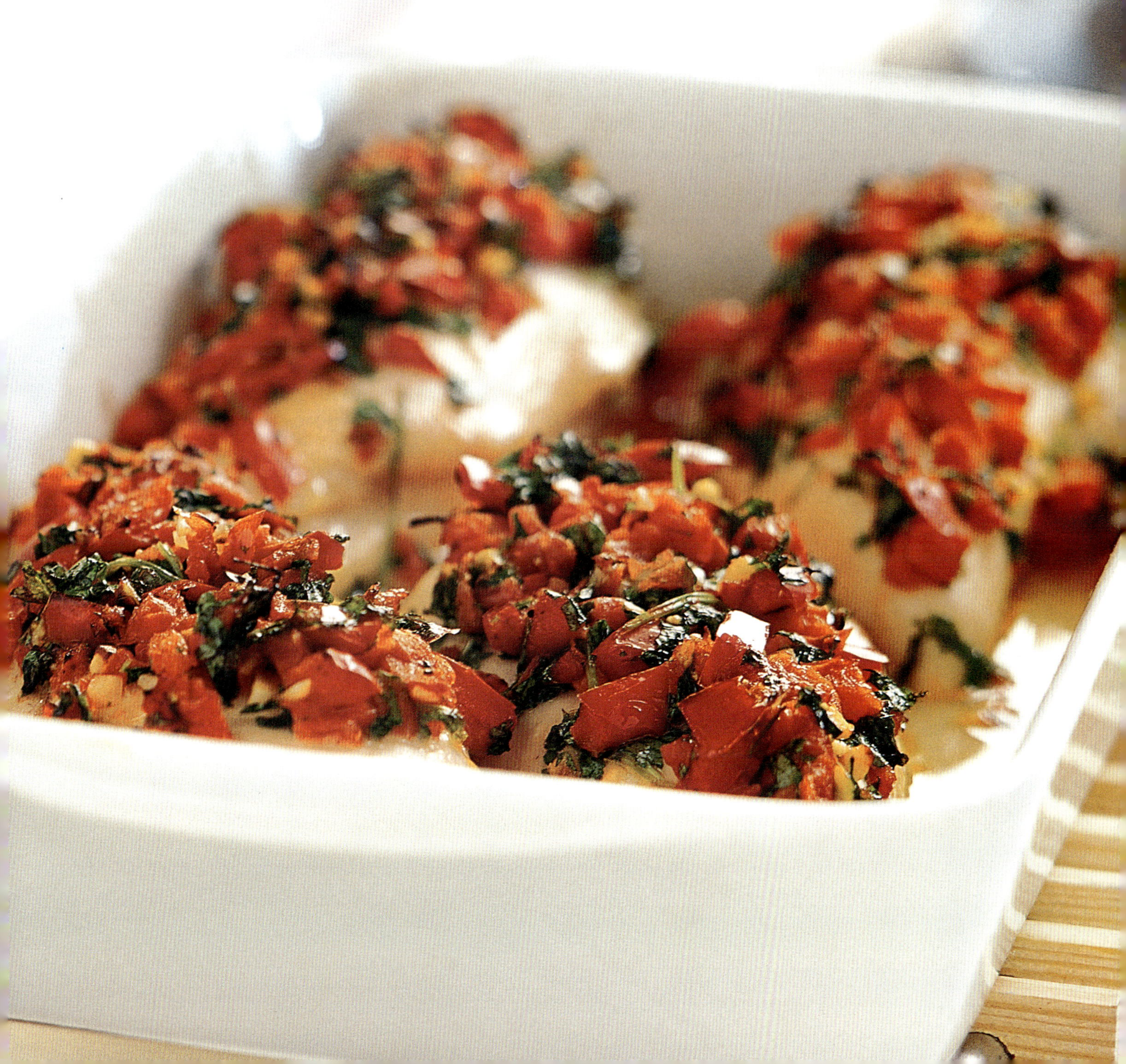

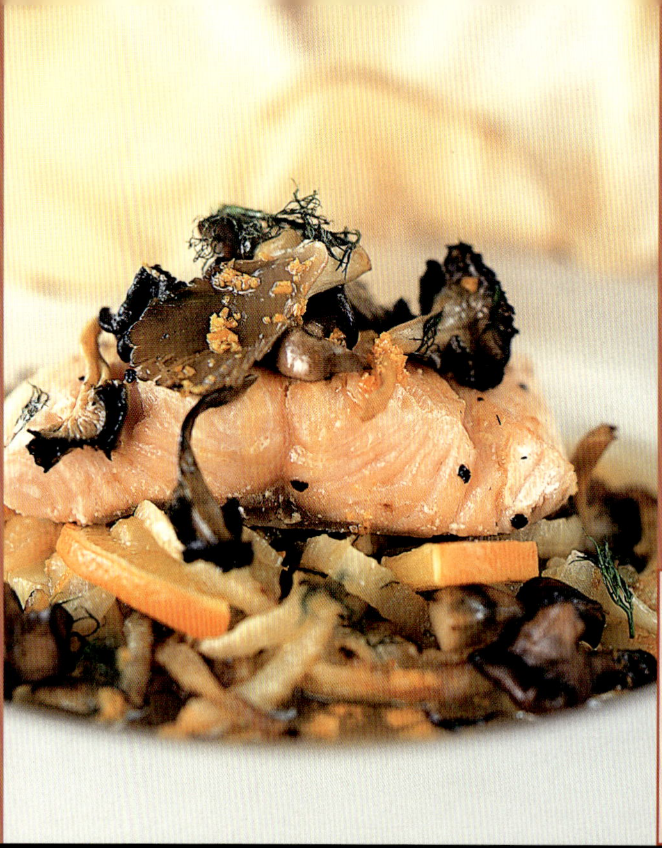

PER SERVING
413 kcalories
protein 32g
carbohydrate 6g
fat 29g
saturated fat 11g
fibre 4g
added sugar none
salt 0.77g

# Alpha plus to the omegas

*The omega-3 oils seem to be something new that we all now have to be conscious of getting in our diet. But what did people do before any of us had heard of them?*

**What exactly are the omega-3 oils?**

*They were at one time better known as polyunsaturated essential fatty acids – of which there are two main families, the omega-6 and the omega-3 fatty acids. The body can make all but two fatty acids – linoleic acid (the principal omega-6) and alpha-linolenic acid (the principal omega-3). Scientists now know that these have different functions in maintaining a healthy body.*

**What are their best sources?**

*Alpha-linolenic acid is mostly found in oils such as flax seed (linseed), soya, walnut and rapeseed oils, also in nuts and seeds. Two other fatty acids known as EPA and DHA can be derived from alpha-linolenic acid, so are not strictly speaking 'essential' (i.e. having to be supplied in our diet). However, they are also found in quantity in oily fish, e.g. salmon, sardines, mackerel, tuna, etc., and fish oils. Even canned fish has useful quantities of the oils, especially if canned in oil rather than brine. The principal essential fatty acids in the omega-6 group are linoleic acid – found in vegetable oils, like sunflower and corn oils, nuts, seeds and leafy vegetables – and arachidonic acid, found in lean meats.*

**Why are they important for us?**

*The essential fatty acids have been found to help combat a wide range of conditions from cancer and arthritis to female reproductive problems. The omega-3 oils are now known to be particularly effective in preventing heart disease and strokes by keeping the blood healthily 'unsticky'. The omega-6 fatty acids also help reduce blood cholesterol levels, especially 'bad' LDLs (see page 94).*

**Due to it now being widely farmed, omega-3-rich salmon is available at most fishmongers and in most supermarkets at very good prices ▶**

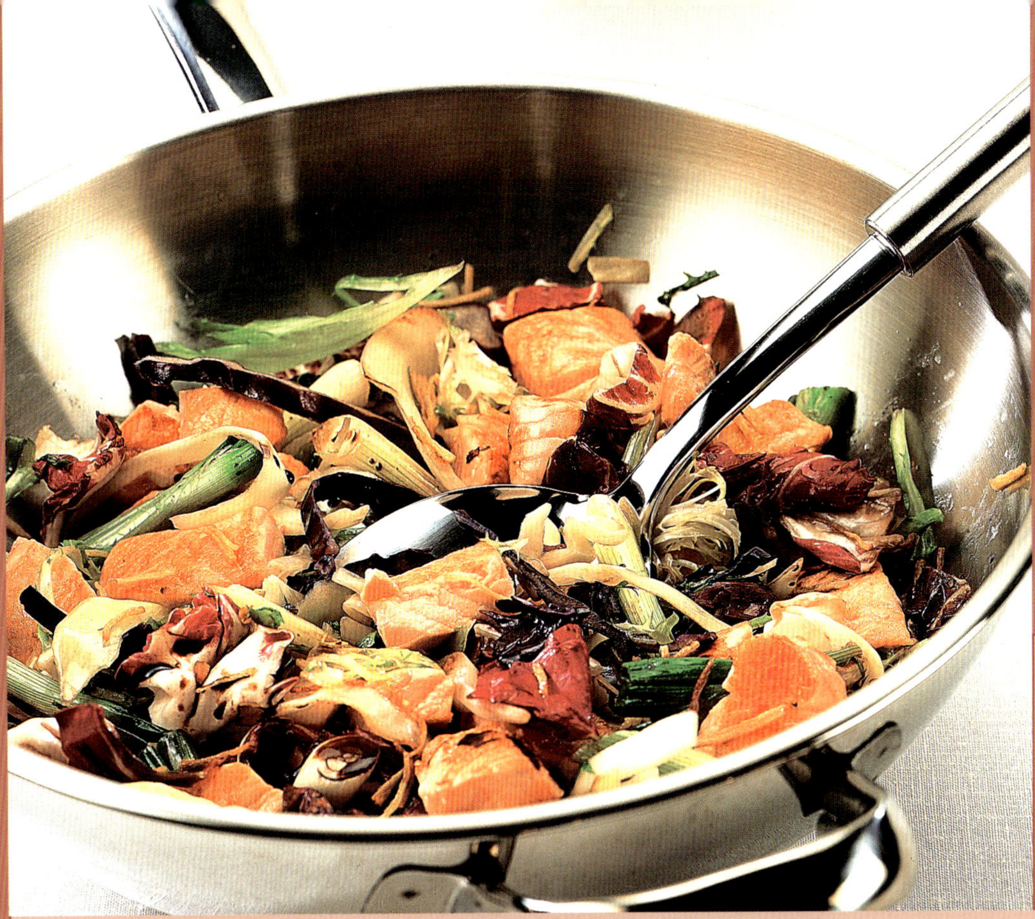

PER SERVING
**248 kcalories**
**protein 24g**
**carbohydrate 3g**
**fat 16g**
**saturated fat 3g**
**fibre 1g**
**added sugar none**
**salt 0.26g**

**Salmon Stir-fry with Wilted Leaves** *(above) starts by heating 1 tablespoon of oil in a frying pan, adding 5cm/2in piece of fresh ginger, grated, and cooking for 30 seconds, stirring. Then season 450g/1lb salmon fillet, skinned and cut into 2.5cm/1in cubes, add to the pan and cook for 5 minutes, turning once until just cooked through and beginning to brown.*

*Remove the salmon from the pan and keep warm. Add 1 bunch of spring onions, cut into 4cm/1½in lengths, and stir-fry for 3–4 minutes until just soft. Pour over 150ml/¼ pint hot vegetable stock and bring to the boil. Tip in 225g/8oz mixed salad leaves and cook for 1 minute to wilt. Tip in 2 tablespoons soy sauce and serve hot from the pan with steamed or boiled rice.*

**Paper-wrapped Salmon with Orange Butter, Fennel and Mushrooms** *(opposite) provides essential fatty acids with a flourish. Preheat the oven to 180°C/350°F/Gas 4. Season 4 skinless salmon fillets, each about 150g/5oz, with salt and pepper. Discard any tough outer leaves from 2–3 fennel bulbs, each about 225g/8oz, then thinly slice, cutting out the core and reserving the feathery fronds. Melt 15g/½oz butter in a frying pan and fry the fennel for about 3–4 minutes until slightly softened and tinged brown, then remove from the pan. Toss in 100g/4oz mixed mushrooms, such as chestnut, cep or girolle, sliced if large, add 15g/½oz more butter and stir briefly to coat.*

*Slice 1 orange and grate the zest from another. Beat the zest into 30g/1oz butter. Cut out four 35cm/14in circles from sheets of non-stick baking parchment or greaseproof paper. Divide the fennel between the circles and tuck in the orange slices. Sprinkle over the fennel fronds. Top with a salmon fillet and scatter over the mushrooms. Season with salt and pepper and put a knob of orange butter on top.*

*Fold the paper over to enclose everything and twist the edges to completely seal. Put each parcel on a baking sheet and bake for 12–15 minutes. Check the fish is cooked (a skewer inserted into the thickest part comes out warm); if not, cook for a few minutes more and retest. Serve in the parcels, so the aroma when opened can be enjoyed at the table, accompanied by new potatoes.*

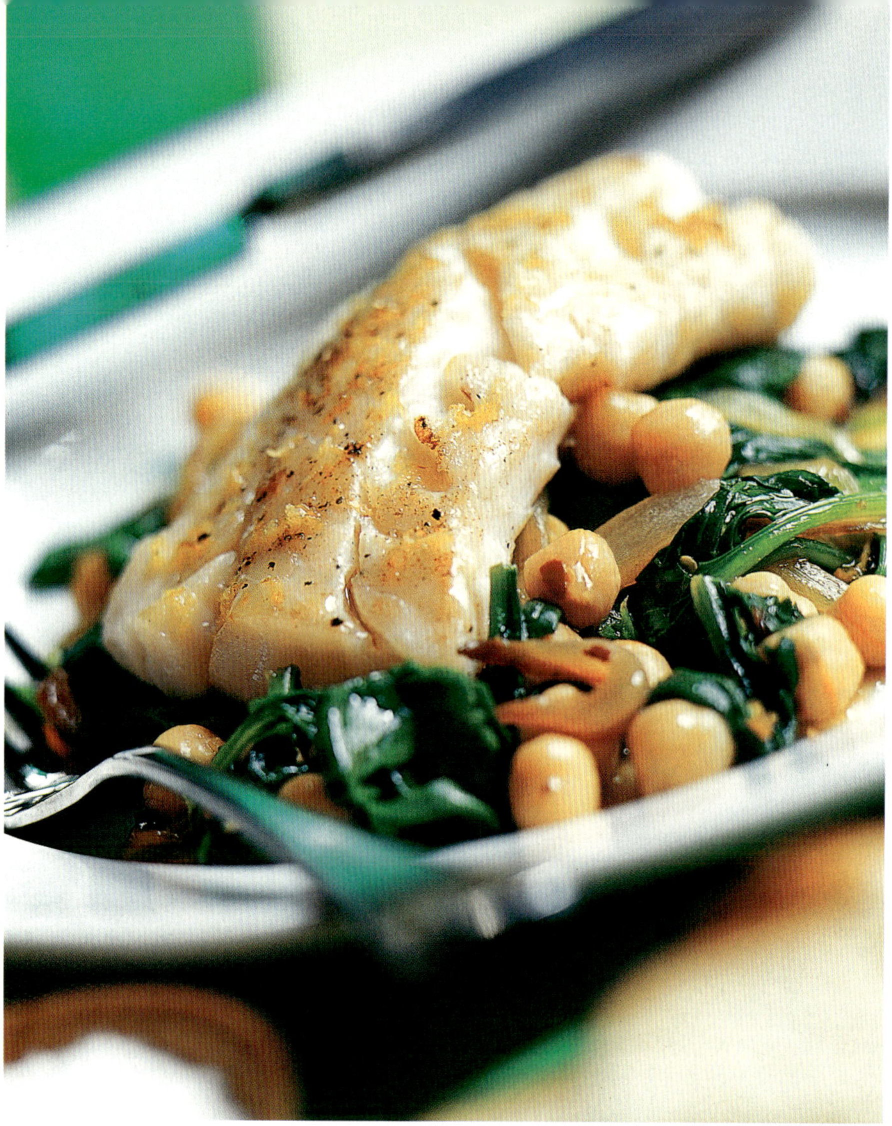

# Lemon Cod with Spicy Chickpeas

PER SERVING
**306 kcalories**
**protein 32g**
**carbohydrate 14g**
**fat 13g**
**saturated fat 2g**
**fibre 4g**
**added sugar none**
**salt 1.03g**

**Chickpeas (even the canned variety) are an excellent source of vitamin E, which is not only great for skin health but is a valuable antioxidant, scouring the body for the damaging free radicals that can cause cancer.**

PREPARATION about 15 minutes
COOKING 8–10 minutes

zest and juice of 1 lemon
3 tbsp light olive oil, plus more for drizzling (optional)
4 skinned cod fillets, each about 150g/5oz
1 onion, sliced into thin wedges
250g/9oz packet of fresh spinach, stems trimmed
½–1 tsp dried chilli flakes
420g/15oz can of chickpeas, rinsed and drained

1 Preheat the grill. Mix the lemon zest with 1 tablespoon of oil. Line a roasting tin with foil, oil lightly and add the fish. Brush the fish with lemon oil. Season and grill for 8–10 minutes until cooked (the foil reflects heat, so there is no need to turn the fish).

2 Meanwhile, heat the rest of the oil in a frying pan and fry the onion until golden. Add the spinach and cook until wilted. Stir in the chilli flakes. Tip in the chickpeas and 1 tablespoon of lemon juice, and heat through.

3 Season and spoon the chickpea mixture on to hot plates. Serve the fish on top, drizzled with a little extra oil or lemon juice.

# Chillied Trout with Chinese Leaves

PER SERVING
391 kcalories
protein 48g
carbohydrate 9g
fat 18g
saturated fat 3g
fibre 1g
added sugar none
salt 4.36g

SERVES 2
PREPARATION 10 minutes
COOKING 8–10 minutes

**Although not quite as rich in the omega-3 oils (page 76) as the really oily fish like salmon, mackerel and sardines, trout is nevertheless a very good source. Steamed rice is all the accompaniment you'll need.**

- 2.5cm/1in piece of fresh root ginger
- 2 rainbow trout, each about 350g/12oz, filleted but with the skin left on
- 2 tbsp groundnut oil
- 3 tbsp dark soy sauce
- 2 garlic cloves, finely chopped
- 1 small hot red chilli, deseeded and finely chopped
- 2 small heads of bok choy or other Chinese leaves (total weight about 200g/7oz), each halved lengthwise
- 1/2 tsp cornflour
- a few drops of dark sesame oil
- a few fresh coriander sprigs, to garnish

1 Slice half the ginger into fine shreds and chop the rest. Season the trout fillets lightly on both sides with salt and pepper. Heat half the oil in a large frying pan over a high heat. Add the trout fillets and sear them for about 30 seconds on each side.

2 Take the frying pan off the heat and add the soy sauce, garlic, chopped ginger and chilli. Reduce the heat to moderate, return the pan to the heat and cook the trout on one side only for 3 minutes, until it is just cooked through.

3 Meanwhile, heat the remaining groundnut oil in a wok or another frying pan and add the shredded ginger. Stir-fry briefly, then add the bok choy or other leaves and stir-fry for a minute or two until just beginning to wilt. Mix the cornflour with 2 teaspoons of cold water, tip in the cornflour mixture with 4 tablespoons of water and stir-fry briefly until bubbling and thickened. Stir in the sesame oil.

4 To serve, divide the greens between 2 warmed plates and place 2 trout fillets on top of each. Drizzle with the liquid, garnish with coriander sprigs and serve immediately.

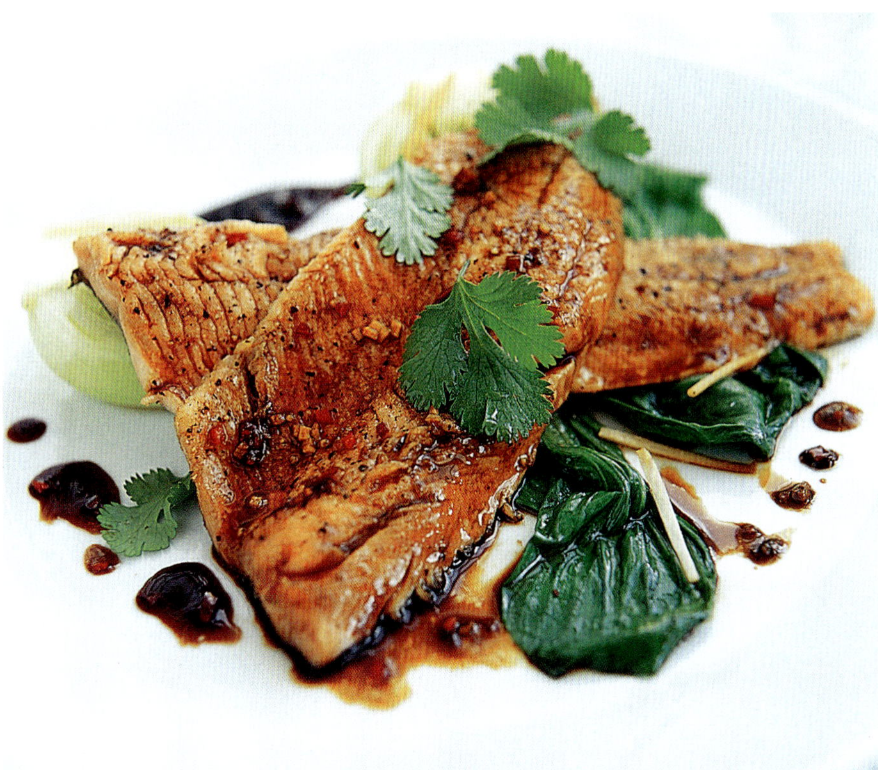

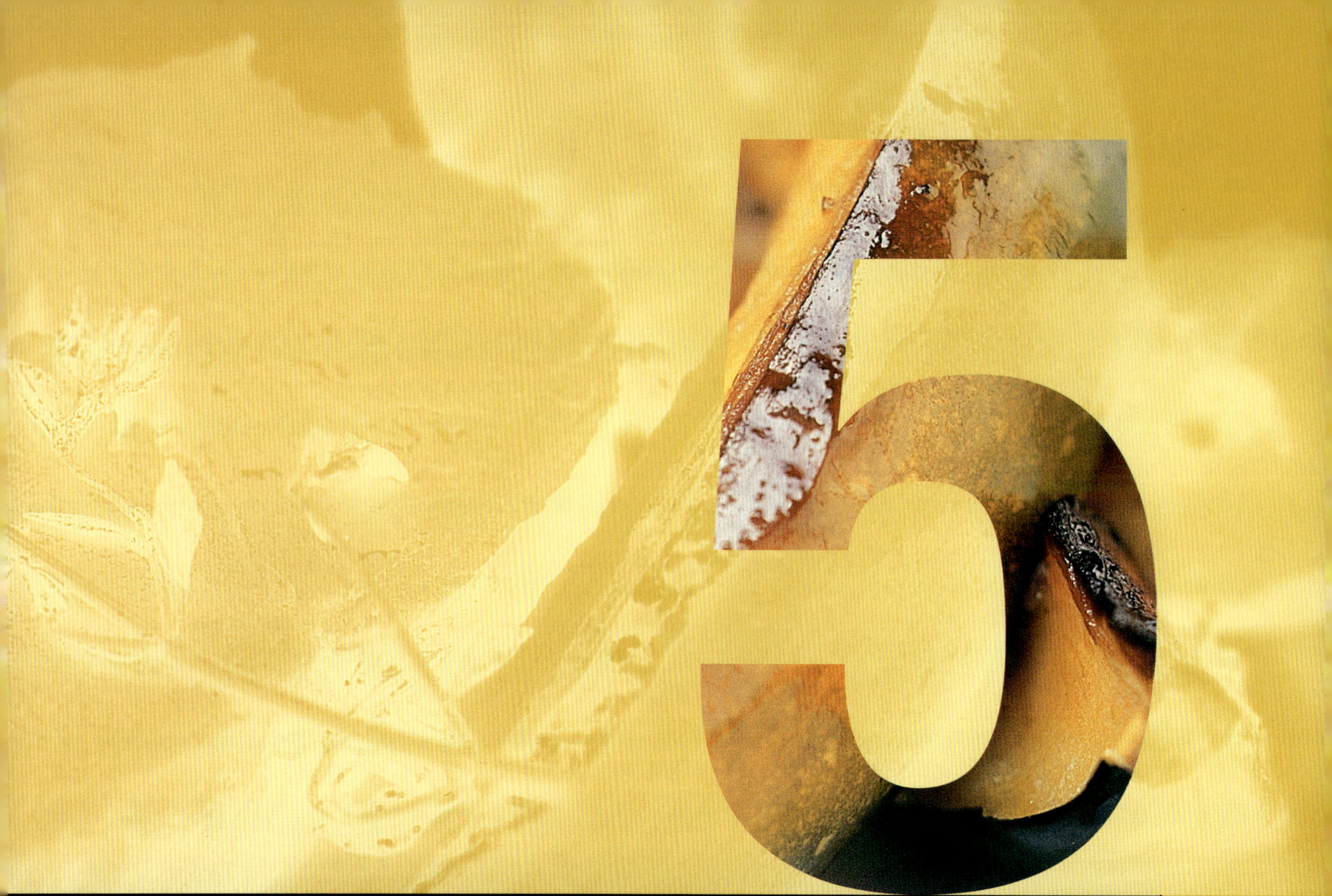

# 5

## Smart Show-off and Party Dishes

*Until quite recently, it was thought that making food for entertaining automatically meant adding lots of rich ingredients, like cream and alcohol – and certainly there was usually great emphasis on lavish use of red meat. Nowadays, however, we have learned that special-occasion dishes can be just as healthy as everyday food without in any way detracting from flavour, visual appeal or 'wow' factor. Of course, some of our best allies in nutritious eating have been eternally popular in party food – like seafood and salmon.*

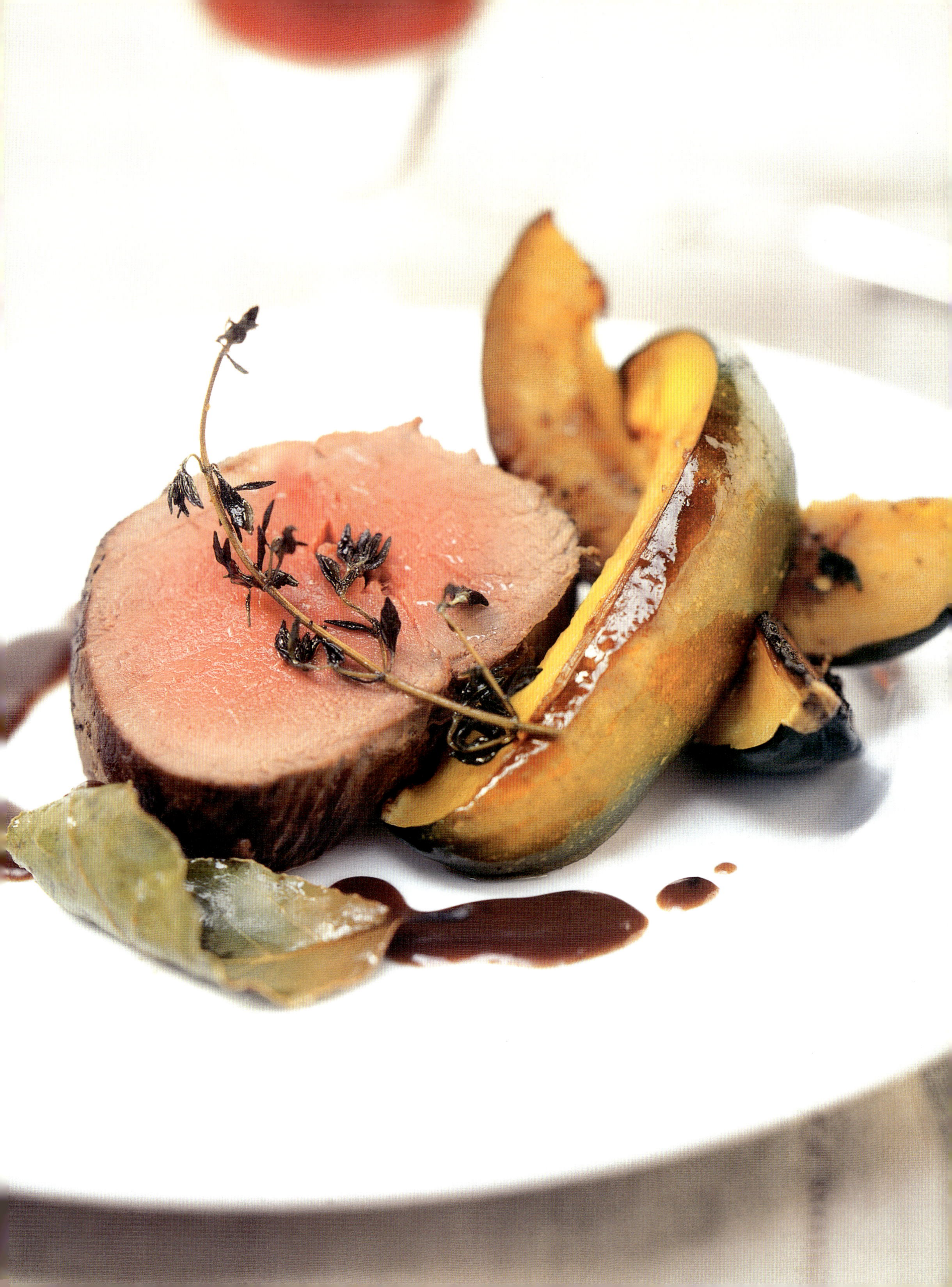

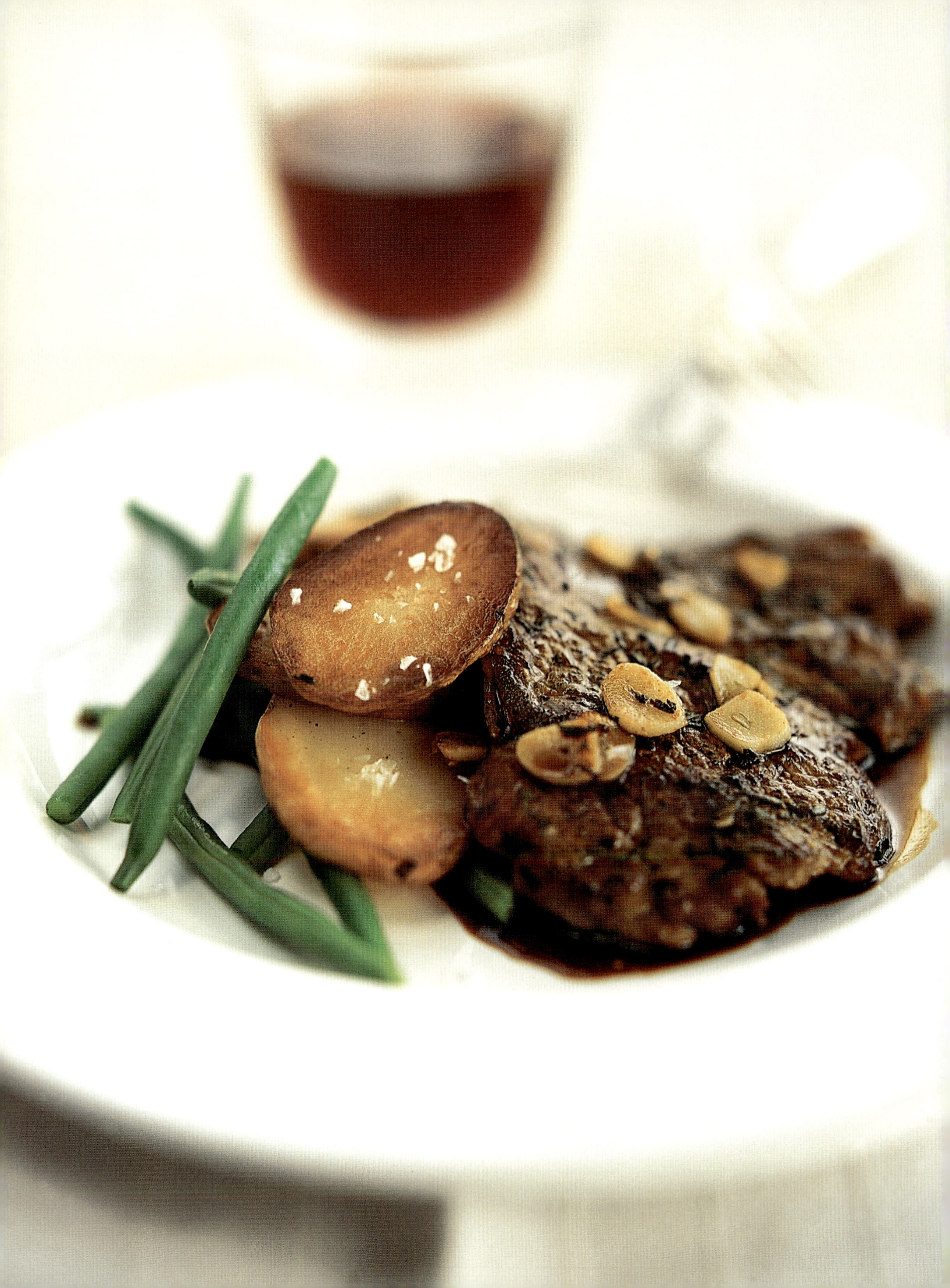

# Venison with Herbed Pumpkin Wedges

**PER SERVING**
378 kcalories
protein 58g
carbohydrate 10g
fat 9g
saturated fat 1g
fibre 2g
added sugar none
salt 0.72g

**Venison is among the healthiest of red meats, with a much lower saturated fat content, closer to that of poultry. It is also full of vitamins and minerals, especially iron.**

SERVES 6
PREPARATION 20 minutes
COOKING 40 minutes

1.5kg/3¼lb piece of venison fillet
3 tbsp olive oil
1.3kg/3lb unpeeled pumpkin
4 bay leaves
5 fresh thyme sprigs
4 shallots, finely chopped
2 garlic cloves, finely chopped
1 tbsp crushed juniper berries
grated zest and juice of 1 orange
150ml/¼ pint port
600ml/1 pint lamb or beef stock
1 tbsp redcurrant jelly
knob of cold butter

1 Preheat the oven to 220°C/425°F/Gas 7. Tie the venison fillet with string at 5cm/2in intervals along its length.
2 Heat a tablespoon of oil in a heavy roasting tin on the hob, then season the meat and fry all over to seal.
3 Cut the pumpkin into wedges, add to the tin and season. Add 3 bay leaves, 3 thyme sprigs and the remaining oil. Turn the wedges in the oil and roast for 30–35 minutes, turning twice, until the meat is slightly pink inside.
4 Put meat and pumpkin on a plate and cover to keep warm. Drain all but a tablespoon of oil from the roasting tin, then add the shallots and garlic. Cook over a moderate heat for 5–7 minutes until the shallots are golden. Add the juniper and orange zest and juice; bubble for 30 seconds. Add the port and remaining bay and thyme, then cook for 5 minutes, stirring occasionally, until reduced by half. Stir in the stock and boil until reduced by half again.
5 Sieve into a clean pan, rubbing gently with the back of a spoon. Return to the heat, add the jelly and stir to melt. Whisk in the butter until thickened and glossy; season. Carve the meat and serve with the sauce and pumpkin.

# Pan-fried Beef with Garlic, Rosemary and Balsamic Vinegar

**PER SERVING**
327 kcalories
protein 40g
carbohydrate 6g
fat 16g
saturated fat 6g
fibre none
added sugar none
salt 0.86g

SERVES 6
PREPARATION 5 minutes
COOKING 15 minutes

6 sirloin steaks, each about 175g/6oz
2 tbsp olive oil
3 garlic cloves, thinly sliced
3 tbsp roughly chopped fresh rosemary
175ml/6fl oz balsamic vinegar
600ml/1 pint beef stock, preferably home-made
sautéed potatoes and steamed green beans, to serve

1 Put the steaks between 2 sheets of film and bat out to a thickness of about 1cm/½in.
2 Heat the olive oil in a large frying pan, then add the garlic and cook until it just begins to sizzle. Remove the garlic with a slotted spoon and allow to drain on kitchen paper.
3 Season the steaks, then top with rosemary and transfer to the pan. Cook for 1–2 minutes on each side for medium-rare steak. Increase the cooking time by another minute or two for a more well-done steak. (You may have to cook the steaks in batches.) Transfer the steaks and rosemary to a plate and keep warm.
4 Pour the vinegar into the pan and bubble rapidly, scraping up any bits from the base of the pan, until reduced by half. Add the beef stock and allow the mixture to bubble for 4 minutes until reduced and slightly syrupy.
5 Transfer the steaks to warm serving plates and pour over the sauce. Scatter the reserved garlic and rosemary over the top of each steak. Serve with sautéed potatoes and green beans.

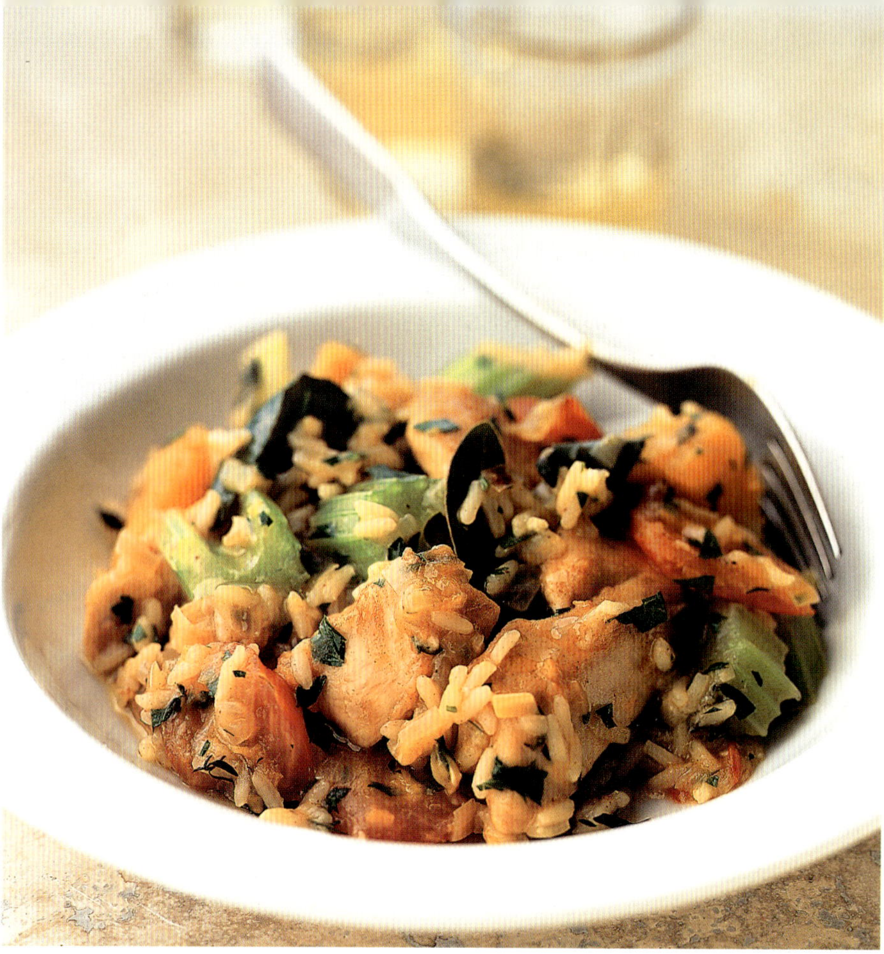

**PER SERVING**
**437 kcalories**
**protein 39g**
**carbohydrate 39g**
**fat 15g**
**saturated fat 3g**
**fibre 4g**
**added sugar none**
**salt 1.45g**

# Chicken and Pumpkin Cajun Gumbo

**Don't remove the bay leaves from this sumptuously flavoured Cajun-style stew – the Cajuns consider them good luck.**

PREPARATION 20 minutes
COOKING 25–30 minutes

4 skinless chicken breast fillets, each about 150g/5oz, roughly chopped
2 tbsp plain flour
1–2 tsp hot chilli powder
2 tsp paprika
3 tbsp olive oil
2 onions, chopped
2 celery stalks, roughly chopped
4 garlic cloves, finely chopped
4 bay leaves
1 tbsp fresh thyme leaves or 1 tsp dried thyme
350g/12oz pumpkin flesh (you'll need 1 whole pumpkin or a slice of pumpkin weighing about 700g/1lb 9oz), cubed
1.3 litres/2¼ pints chicken stock
175g/6oz long-grain rice
8 small tomatoes, deseeded and chopped
3 tbsp chopped fresh parsley

1 Toss the chicken in the flour, chilli powder and paprika. Cover and set aside.
2 Heat the oil in a large pan, then cook the onions, celery and garlic for 3–4 minutes until the onion has softened. Remove the onion mixture from the pan and set aside.
3 Cook the chicken, flour and spices in the pan for 6–7 minutes, turning occasionally, until the chicken is browned on all sides.
4 Return the onion mixture to the pan with the bay, thyme and pumpkin. Add the stock and season. Cover and simmer gently for 15 minutes.
5 Add the rice; stir once and simmer uncovered for 15–20 minutes until the rice is tender.
6 Stir in the tomatoes and parsley, heat through for 2 minutes, season and serve.

# Glazed Duck with Pasta Ribbons

PER SERVING
478 kcalories
protein 32g
carbohydrate 69g
fat 10g
saturated fat 2g
fibre 5g
added sugar 4g
salt 0.36g

**Duck is thought of as being very high in fat content, but it needn't be, so long as you remove the skin and cook the meat with care. In this recipe, the duck is kept moist by roasting it in its orange marinade. Pappardelle are broad flat noodles (the name means 'gulp down pasta'), available with plain or frilled edges. In Italy, they are a traditional accompaniment to many game dishes, while most large supermarkets over here now stock them. Asparagus is a 'superfood' (see page 100) and a good source of folic acid.**

PREPARATION 15 minutes
COOKING 30 minutes

1 tbsp clear honey
1 tbsp white wine vinegar
2 tsp tomato purée
grated zest and juice of 1 orange
two 225g/8oz duck breast fillets, skinned
8 plum tomatoes, halved lengthwise
300g/10oz pappardelle or tagliatelle pasta
225g/8oz thin asparagus, cut into 2.5cm/1in lengths

**to serve**
2 tsp olive oil
2 tbsp shredded fresh basil
2 tbsp freshly grated Parmesan cheese

1 Preheat the oven to 200°C/400°F/Gas 6. In a bowl, mix together the honey, vinegar, tomato purée and orange zest. Brush this over the duck and put it in a large roasting tin. Arrange the tomatoes, cut-side up, around the duck. Pour over the orange juice, season and roast for 30 minutes, until the tomatoes and duck are browned and tender.

2 Meanwhile, cook the pasta in a large pan of boiling salted water according to the packet instructions, until tender but still firm to the bite. Add the asparagus about 3 minutes before the end of cooking time.

3 Remove the roasting tin from the oven and let the duck rest for 5 minutes. Cut each breast across into 1cm/½in wide strips and return to the roasting tin with the juices.

4 Drain the pasta and asparagus, tip into the roasting tin and toss together with the duck strips. Divide between warm plates, drizzle over the olive oil and scatter with basil and Parmesan.

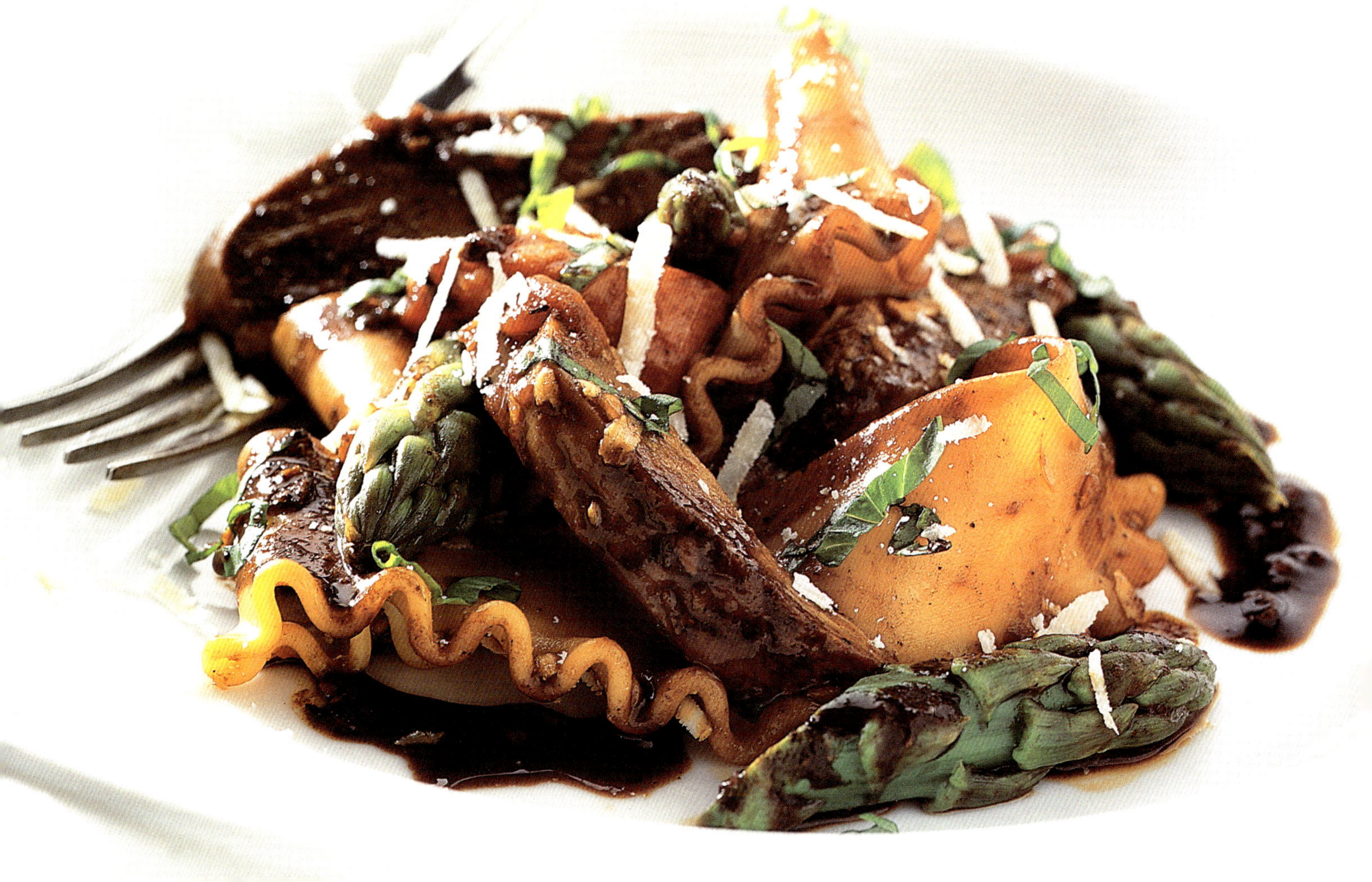

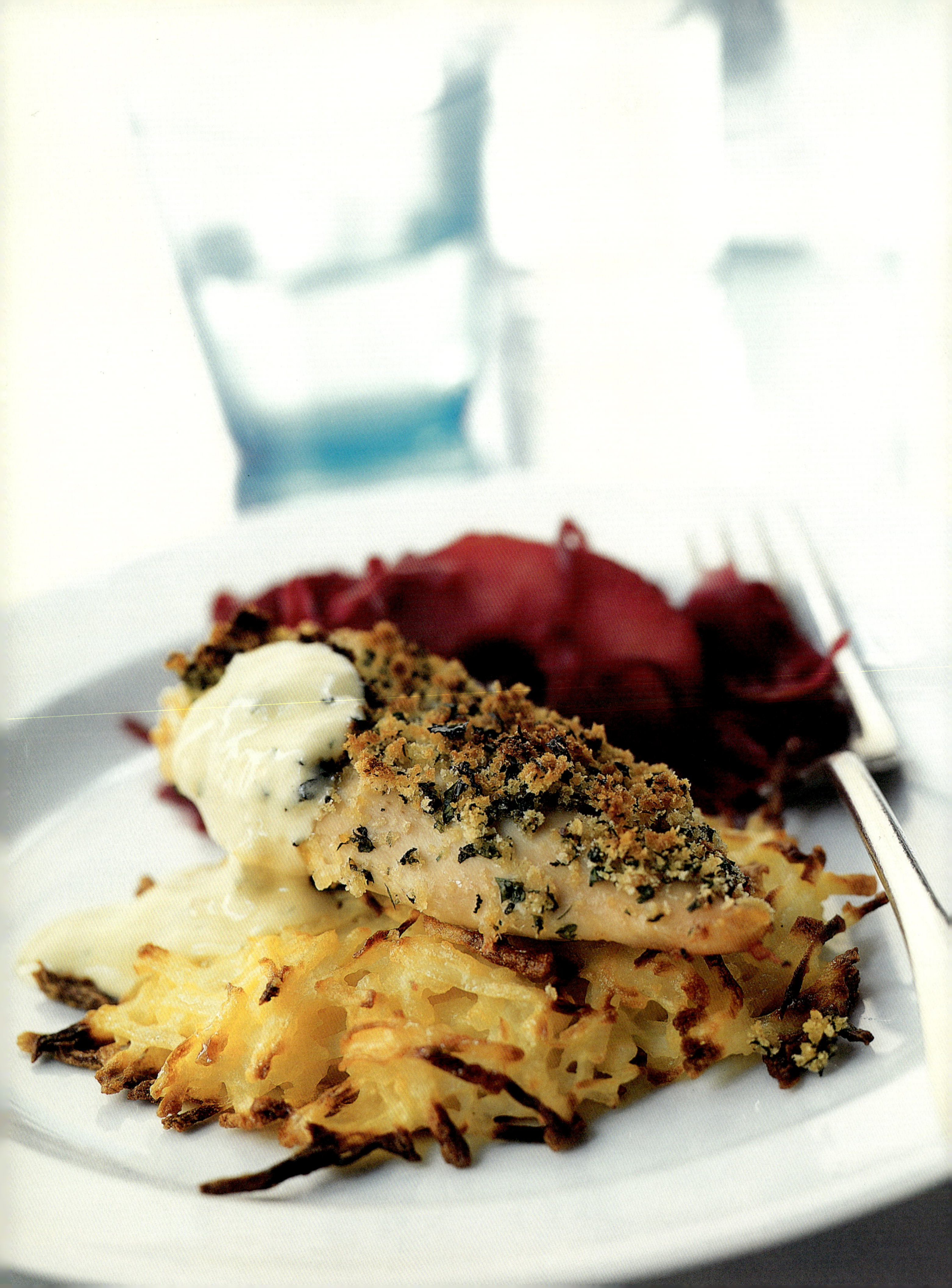

# Rösti Chicken Breasts with Red Cabbage

**Using stale bread for the breadcrumbs gives a crunchier result. Red cabbage has much the same nutritional content as green cabbage.**

**PER SERVING**
**464 kcalories**
**protein 41g**
**carbohydrate 45g**
**fat 13g**
**saturated fat 4g**
**fibre 5g**
**added sugar 5g**
**salt 0.94g**

PREPARATION 30 minutes
COOKING 40–45 minutes

- 1 tbsp olive oil
- 500g/1lb 2oz potatoes, such as Estima or Maris Piper
- 1 garlic clove, finely chopped
- 1 small egg, beaten
- 4 tbsp white breadcrumbs
- 1 tbsp chopped fresh parsley, plus more to garnish
- 1 tbsp chopped fresh sage leaves
- 1 tsp finely grated lemon zest
- 4 skinless chicken breast fillets, each about 150g/5oz
- 225g/8oz red cabbage, shredded
- 1 eating apple, peeled, cored and sliced
- 1 tbsp fresh lemon juice
- 2 tsp light muscovado sugar
- 4 tbsp port or red wine
- 4 tbsp half-fat crème fraîche

1 Preheat the oven to 190°C/375°F/Gas 5. Grease a small roasting tin and a baking sheet with 1 teaspoon of the olive oil.

2 Cook the potatoes in boiling salted water for 10 minutes, then drain. Leave until cool enough to handle, then grate coarsely.

3 In a bowl, mix the grated potatoes with the garlic, beaten egg and plenty of salt and pepper. Pile into 4 mounds on the baking sheet and flatten slightly into cakes.

4 Mix the breadcrumbs, herbs and lemon zest with another teaspoon of the olive oil, then season. Sit the chicken breasts in the roasting tin and sprinkle over the breadcrumb mixture.

5 Bake for 10 minutes, then put the potato cakes in the oven with the chicken and bake for a further 20 minutes until the chicken is cooked and the topping golden.

6 About 10 minutes before the end of cooking time, put the cabbage in a pan with the apple, lemon juice, sugar and port or red wine. Season with salt and pepper. Cover and cook for 8–10 minutes over a low heat, stirring occasionally until tender.

7 Divide the potato röstis between 4 plates. Lay a chicken breast on top of each, put a spoonful of red cabbage by the side and keep warm.

8 Add the crème fraîche to the meat juices in the roasting tin and stir over a gentle heat to make a sauce. Drizzle over the chicken and around the cabbage. Sprinkle over the parsley and serve.

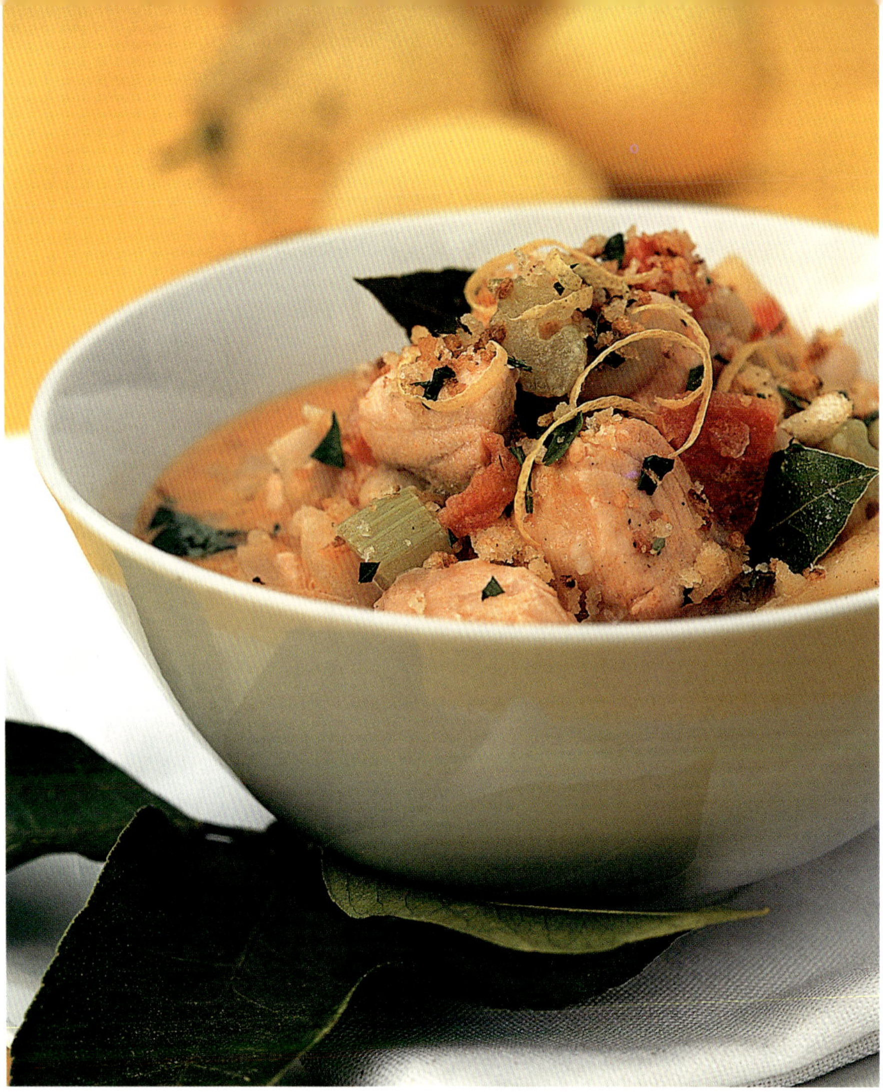

**PER SERVING**
429 kcalories
protein 31g
carbohydrate 25g
fat 23g
saturated fat 7g
fibre 5g
added sugar none
salt 1.2g

# Salmon, Cannellini and Lemon Crumb Stew

**Fortunately, ready-cooked pulses canned in brine have much the same nutritional goodness as cooked dried pulses.**

PREPARATION 20 minutes
COOKING 40 minutes

2 lemons
35g/1 1/4oz butter
1 tbsp olive oil
1 onion, finely chopped
2 celery stalks, thinly sliced
2 bay leaves
227g/8oz can of chopped tomatoes
450ml/3/4 pint vegetable stock
400g/14oz can of cannellini beans, drained
450g/1lb salmon fillet, skinned and cut into 2.5cm/1in cubes
3 tbsp fresh white breadcrumbs
2 tbsp chopped fresh parsley

1 Grate the zest from 1 lemon and shred a few strips from the other; squeeze the juice from both.

2 Heat 15g/1/2 oz of the butter with the oil in a large pan and fry the onion and celery for 10 minutes until softened. Stir in the bay leaves, tomatoes and stock, season and simmer uncovered for 20 minutes. Stir in the lemon juice, beans and salmon, and simmer for 8–10 minutes until the salmon is just cooked.

3 Meanwhile, heat the remaining butter in a pan and fry the breadcrumbs for a few minutes until crisp and golden. Stir in the grated zest and parsley. Spoon the stew into bowls, sprinkle over the crumbs and garnish with strips of zest.

# Salmon with Spring Onions and Sizzled Garlic

PREPARATION 5–10 minutes
COOKING 7–9 minutes

4 salmon fillets
1 tbsp groundnut oil or light olive oil
4 tsp light soy sauce
3 spring onions
2 garlic cloves
Chinese noodles or new potatoes, to serve

1 Preheat a moderate-to-hot grill. Brush the salmon lightly with oil and season. Line the grill pan with foil and brush lightly with a little more oil, then lay the fillets skin-side down on it. Sprinkle a teaspoon of soy sauce over each.
2 Grill the salmon on one side only until the flesh is lightly browned and firm to the touch (6–8 minutes). It should be a little less well done in the centre – the flesh there should be a darker pink, and firmer – otherwise it will be dry.
3 Meanwhile, shred the spring onions into long thin strips. Peel the garlic and cut into very thin slices.
4 When the salmon is cooked, quickly heat the remaining oil in a pan, throw in the garlic and fry quickly, stirring, until it starts to turn golden (about 30 seconds).
5 Transfer salmon and juices to warmed plates, scatter over the spring onion strips and quickly spoon over some sizzled garlic. Serve at once with noodles or new potatoes.

PER SERVING
**234 kcalories**
**protein 23g**
**carbohydrate 1g**
**fat 15g**
**saturated fat 3g**
**fibre trace**
**added sugar none**
**salt 1.03g**

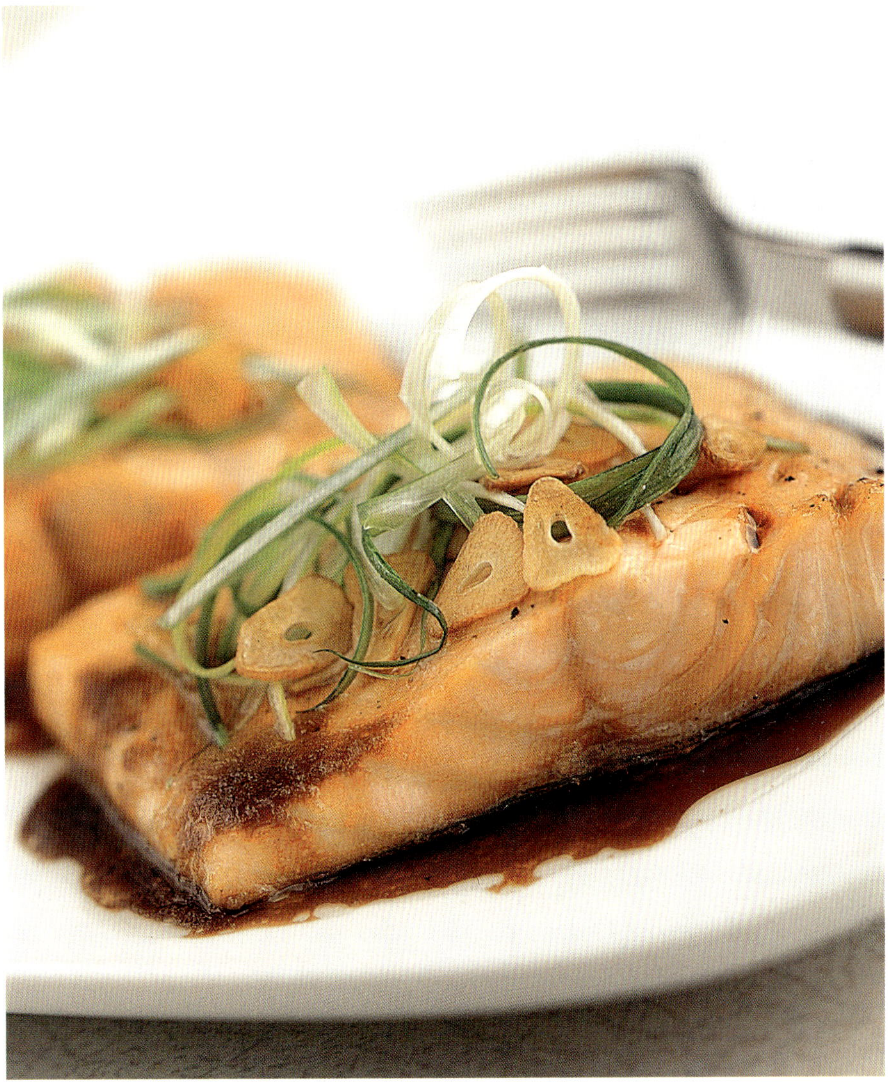

# Cod with Pesto and Potato Slices

**PER SERVING**
**341 kcalories**
**protein 34g**
**carbohydrate 17g**
**fat 16g**
**saturated fat 5g**
**fibre 2g**
**added sugar none**
**salt 0.72g**

**Unless battered and fried, when its level of saturates can multiply horrifically, white fish is a good low-fat source of protein and is packed full of vitamins and minerals.**

PREPARATION 10 minutes
COOKING 30–40 minutes

- 350g/12oz small waxy potatoes (like Maris Piper or Estima), thinly sliced (no need to peel)
- 30g/1oz melted butter
- 4 skinned cod fillets, each about 175g/6oz
- 6 tsp pesto
- 4 tomatoes, halved

1 Preheat the oven to 200°C/400°F/Gas 6. Cook the potatoes in boiling salted water for 7–10 minutes until tender. Drain well, then allow to cool.
2 Brush a shallow ovenproof dish with a little of the butter. Set the fish fillets in the dish in one layer, then sprinkle with salt and pepper. Spread a teaspoon of pesto over each fillet. Arrange the potato slices, overlapping, over the fillets to cover them completely, then season.
3 Arrange the tomato halves, cut side up, around the fish. Smear a little pesto over each cut tomato, then brush the potato slices with the remaining melted butter.
4 Bake for 15–20 minutes until the potatoes are crisp and golden and the fish is tender. Serve hot with a green vegetable (broccoli or green beans go well with this dish).

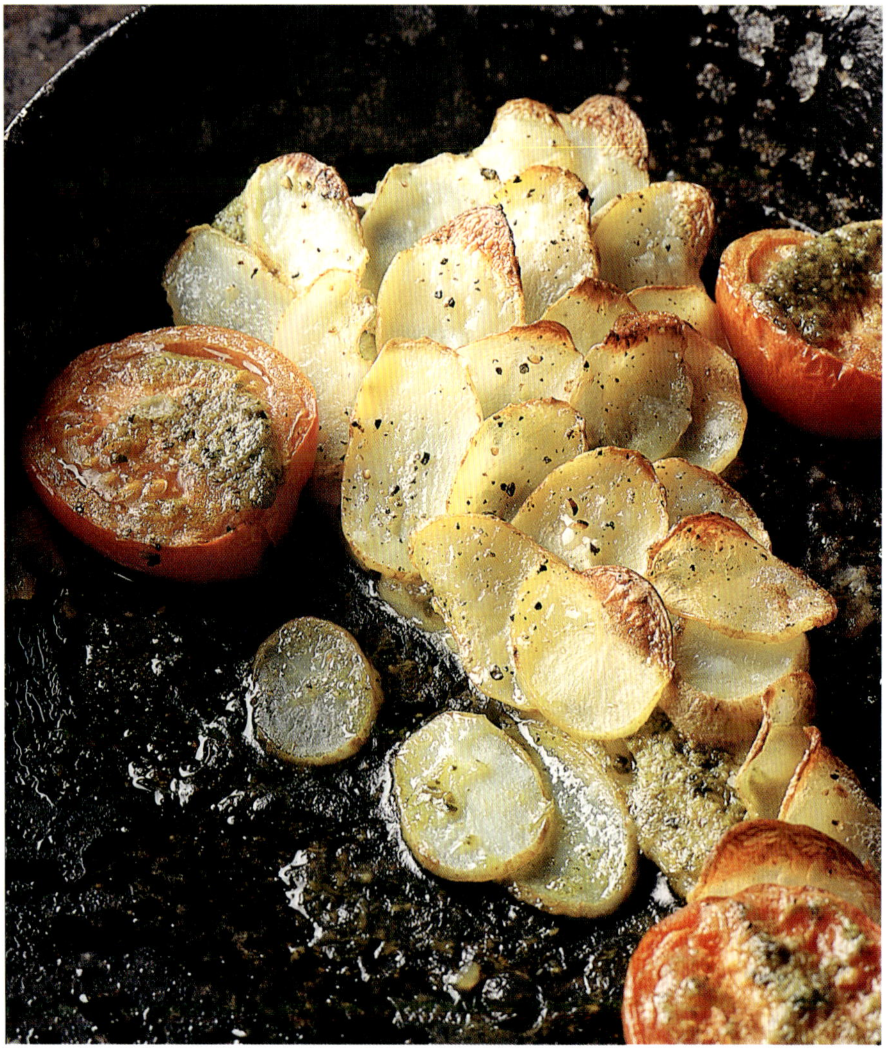

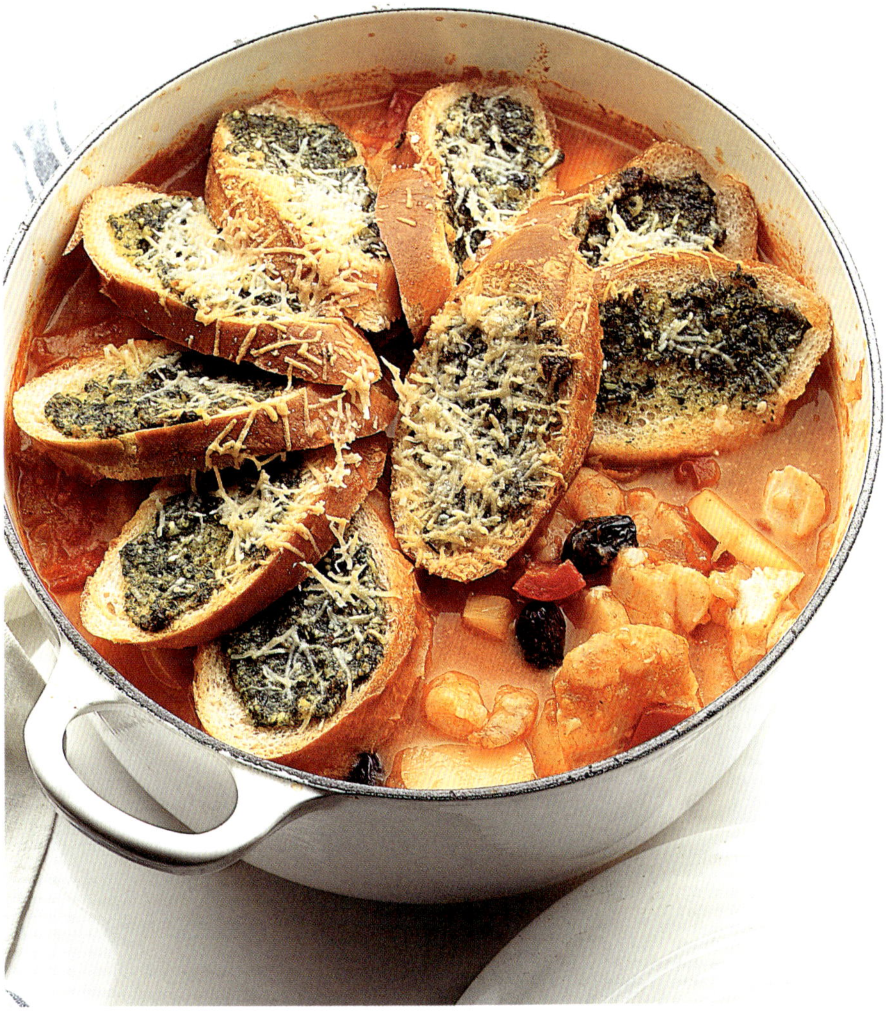

PER SERVING
**435 kcalories**
**protein 41g**
**carbohydrate 34g**
**fat 13g**
**saturated fat 3g**
**fibre 3g**
**added sugar none**
**salt 2.17g**

# Cod and Prawn Casserole with Pesto Toasts

SERVES 6
PREPARATION about 25 minutes
COOKING about 1 hour

450g/1lb ripe tomatoes
2 tbsp olive oil
1 onion, finely chopped
2 garlic cloves, chopped
1 red pepper, cored, deseeded and chopped into small pieces
350g/12oz new potatoes, cut into thick slices
300ml/½ pint white wine
900g/2lb cod, cut into chunks
225g/8oz large peeled cooked prawns
100g/4oz black olives
1 French stick, cut at an angle into 12 slices
2 tbsp pesto
3 tbsp grated Parmesan cheese

VARIATIONS
Simply substitute sun-dried tomato paste or wholegrain mustard for the pesto.

1 Cut around the core of each tomato with the point of a sharp knife, then plunge them into a pan of boiling water. Leave for 30 seconds, then drain. When cool enough to handle, remove the skins and cut the flesh into quarters.
2 Heat the oil in a large frying pan, then fry the onion for 10 minutes until very soft and lightly browned. Add the garlic and red pepper and fry for 5 minutes more. Add the tomatoes, potatoes and wine, and season. Bring to the boil, cover and simmer for 25–30 minutes until the potatoes are tender. Preheat the oven to 200°C/400°F/Gas 6.
3 Remove the pan from the heat and stir in the cod, prawns and olives. Tip into a casserole or other ovenproof dish (about 1.7 litre/3 pint in capacity). Spread one side of each bread slice with pesto, then arrange them overlapping, pesto-side up, on top of the fish.
4 Sprinkle with Parmesan and bake for 25 minutes until the bread is crisp and the cheese has melted.

# Filo Trout Tartlets with Broccoli Stir-fry

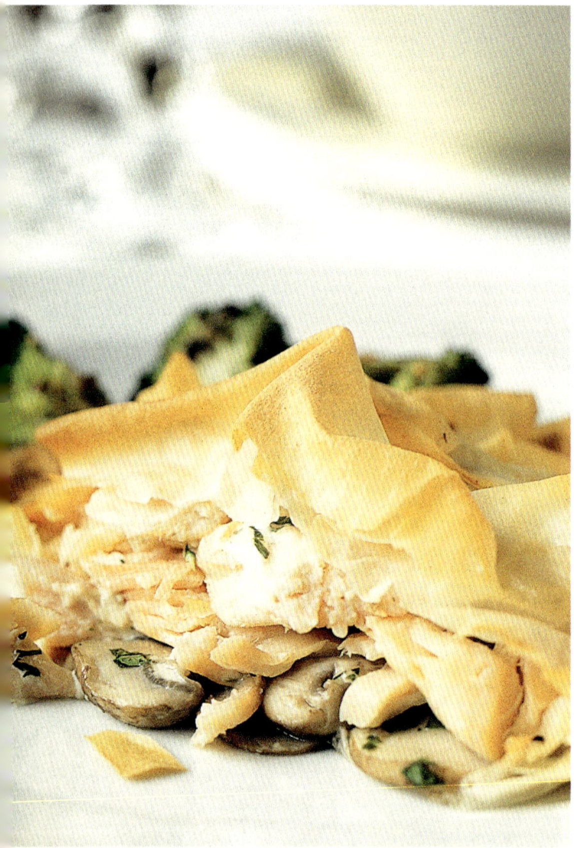

**A great low-fat accompaniment for these trout tartlets is a sauce made by mixing low-fat mayonnaise with lemon juice and mustard.**

PREPARATION 30 minutes
COOKING 15 minutes

2 tbsp olive oil, plus more for brushing
2 garlic cloves, finely chopped
225g/8oz chestnut mushrooms, thinly sliced
2 tbsp finely chopped fresh parsley
8 sheets of filo pastry, each about 31x19cm/12½x7½in
2 tbsp reduced-fat mayonnaise
4 skinless smoked trout fillets, each about 75g/2½oz
1 tsp mustard seeds (optional)
1 small red chilli, deseeded and finely chopped
450g/1lb small broccoli florets
1 tbsp snipped fresh chives

**PER SERVING**
**455 kcalories • protein 30g • carbohydrate 57g fat 13g • saturated fat 2g • fibre 3g added sugar 3g • salt 2.44g**

1 Preheat the oven to 220°C/425°F/Gas 7. Heat half the oil in a frying pan and cook garlic and mushrooms for 4–5 minutes until lightly browned. Season, stir in the parsley and let cool.
2 Cut two 14cm/5½in squares out of each pastry sheet. Line each of 4 muffin or Yorkshire pudding tins with 3 overlapping squares. Spoon mushrooms into the cases, dot with mayonnaise and flake fish on top. Lightly brush remaining squares with olive oil and place one on top of each tartlet, scrunching it to enclose the filling.
3 Bake for 12–15 minutes until the pastry is crisp and golden brown.
4 Meanwhile, heat remaining oil in the pan. Add mustard seeds (if using), chilli and broccoli and cook over high heat for 4–5 minutes until just tender. Season and sprinkle with chives.
5 Serve the tartlets with the broccoli.

# Warm Potato, Mussel and Squid Salad

**PER SERVING**
**515 kcalories**
**protein 46g**
**carbohydrate 37g**
**fat 21g**
**saturated fat 3g**
**fibre 2g**
**added sugar none**
**salt 2.34g**

**Mussels are deemed a 'superfood' (page 100), with all the fantastic B vitamin and mineral content of shellfish coupled with some omega-3 oils (see page 76).**

PREPARATION about 30 minutes
COOKING about 15 minutes, plus cooling

1.1kg/2½lb mussels, washed and scrubbed (discarding any that don't close on being tapped)
4 tbsp water
225g/8oz squid, cleaned and prepared
900g/2lb medium salad potatoes, scrubbed or peeled
1½ tbsp white wine or rice vinegar
6 tbsp extra-virgin olive oil
3 heaped tbsp coarsely chopped fresh parsley

1 Put mussels in a large pan with the water, cover and cook on a high heat for 4–5 minutes, shaking occasionally until they open. Strain juices into a bowl; let mussels cool.
2 Shell all but a handful of mussels, discarding any unopened. Slice the squid pouches into rings and cut the tentacles from the heads above the eyes, removing beaks.
3 In a large pan of boiling salted water, cook the potatoes until tender. Drain and leave to cool for 5 minutes.
4 Meanwhile, strain the mussel liquor into a small pan, bring to the boil and reduce by half. In a small bowl, whisk the vinegar with a little black pepper, then stir in the oil.
5 Slice potatoes into a dish. Add squid to mussel juice and poach for 30 seconds. Add all the mussels and cook for 30 seconds. Remove squid and mussels and add to potatoes.
6 Stir the dressing into the mussel juice, spoon over the salad, scatter over parsley and serve immediately.

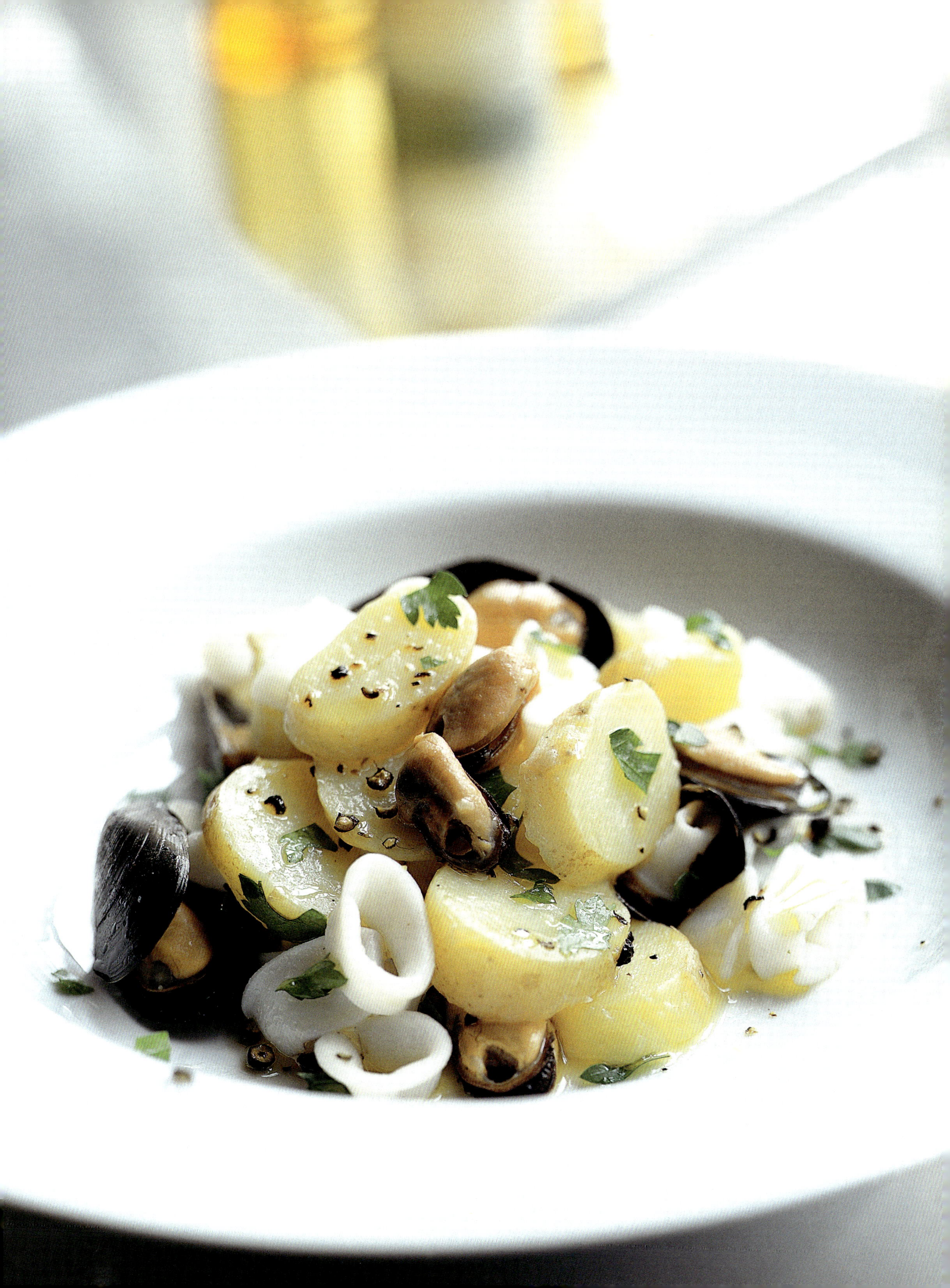

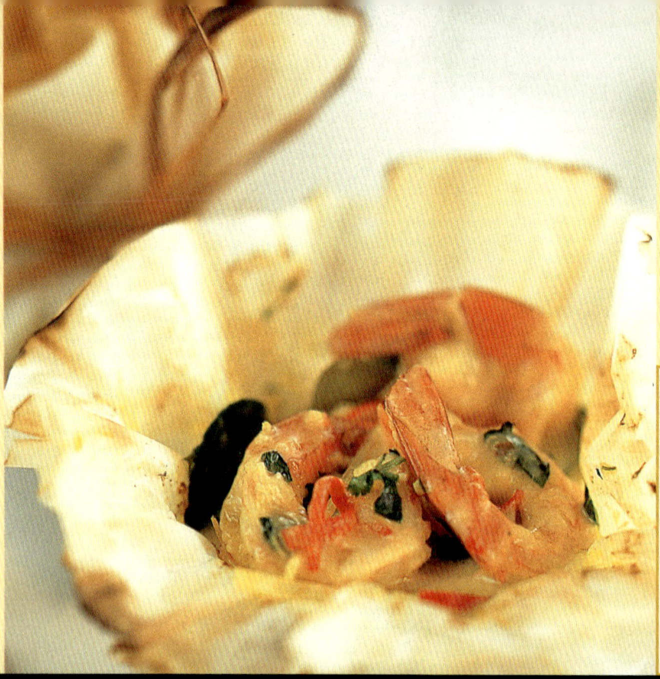

PER SERVING
(for 4)
108 kcalories
protein 19g
carbohydrate 6g
fat 1g
saturated fat trace
fibre trace
added sugar none
salt 0.77g

# All that's good and bad about cholesterol

**Should we worry about cholesterol intake?**

*Possibly even more than fat, cholesterol has often been portrayed as the greatest 'demon' in our food, although nowadays talk is of 'good' and 'bad' cholesterol, so what is the whole story?*

**What exactly is cholesterol?**

*Cholesterol is a white crystalline substance found throughout the body, especially in fats and the blood. It forms an integral part of all cell membranes and the starting point for steroid hormones, including the sex hormones. The body makes about 75% of the cholesterol it needs, and it is broken down by the liver into bile salts, which are involved in fat absorption in the digestive system. It is an essential component of lipoproteins, which transport fats and fatty acids in the blood.*

**'Good' and 'bad' cholesterol**

*High blood levels of low-density lipoprotein cholesterol (LDL-cholesterol or 'bad cholesterol') can get deposited on artery walls, causing hardening. In contrast, high-density lipoprotein cholesterol (HDL-cholesterol or 'good cholesterol') acts as a scavenger, transporting fat and cholesterol to the liver to be broken down.*

**So what can we do?**

*Under normal circumstances, the healthy body regulates its own levels of blood cholesterol. One of the things most likely to upset this balance, however, is a high input of saturated fats, which leads to a surplus of 'bad cholesterol'. Levels of good HDL-cholesterol can, on the other hand, be increased by exercise.*

**The cholesterol in our food**

*The main dietary sources of cholesterol include egg yolks, meat (notably liver) and poultry, seafood (especially shellfish) and dairy produce. Plant products, like fruit, vegetables, pulses and grains, generally contain no cholesterol at all. Normally, though, you needn't worry too much about eating foods that are high in cholesterol, as long as they are part of a balanced diet and you aren't also consuming too much saturated fat.*

**For instance, shellfish can be fairly high in cholesterol, but it is also usually low in fat and full of good nutrients, especially the antioxidants vitamin E and selenium ▶**

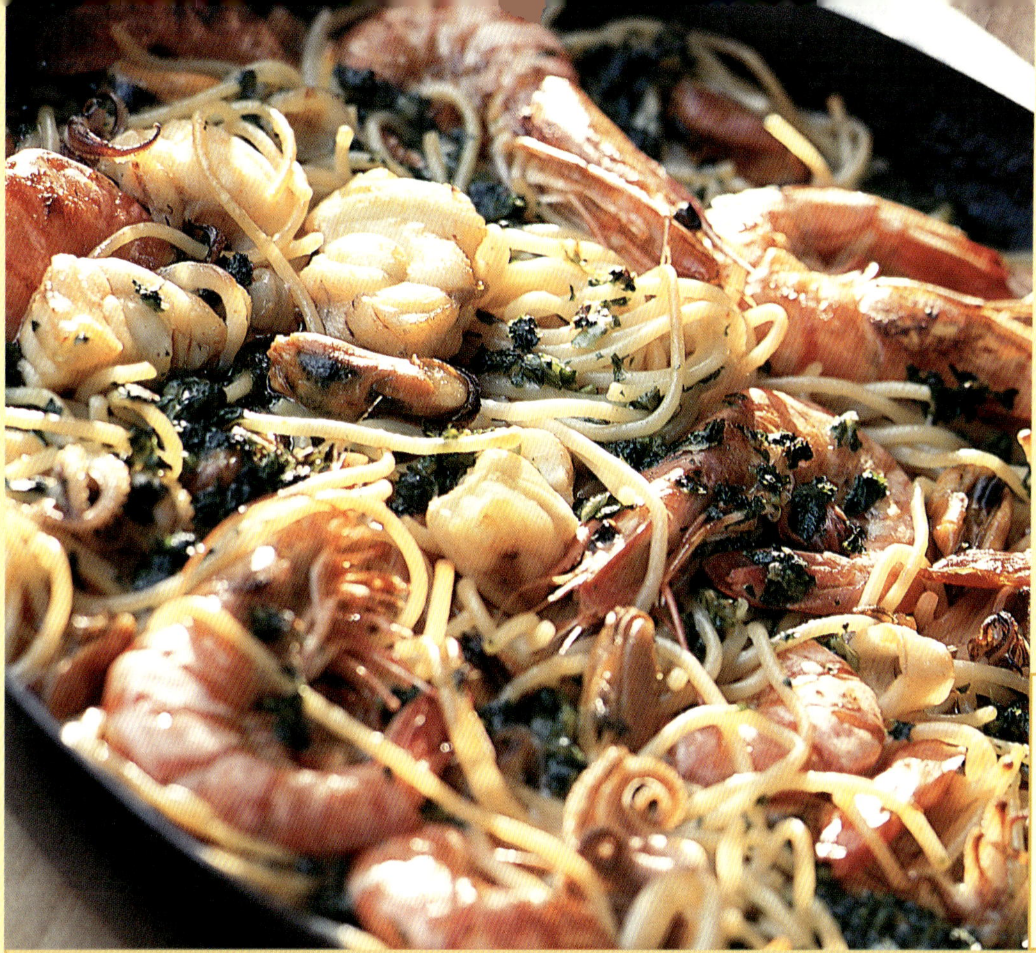

PER SERVING
529 kcalories
protein 39g
carbohydrate 87g
fat 10g
saturated fat 1g
fibre 7g
added sugar none
salt 3.97g

**Seafood Pasta** *(above), for instance, is a very healthy dish with little or no saturated fat. For 6 people, heat 100ml/3½fl oz olive oil in a paella or other wide pan. Clean 300g/10oz squid, cut it into rings, reserving tentacles; cut 350g/12oz skinless monkfish fillets into chunks. Cook these in the oil for 5 minutes. Stir in 2 chopped garlic cloves, a large skinned and finely chopped tomato, ½ teaspoon paprika and some salt. Cook gently for 5 minutes. Add 18 raw tiger prawns in the shell and 12 shelled cooked mussels, then simmer for 3–4 minutes. Add 300g/10oz spaghetti, broken in half, and 1.7 litres/3 pints hot fish stock. Bring to the boil and simmer, uncovered and skimming, for about 10 minutes until the pasta is cooked.*

*Meanwhile, preheat a hot grill and make a picada dressing: pound together 2 garlic cloves and 3 tablespoons chopped parsley. Stir this in, then grill for 5 minutes to crisp the surface slightly.*

**Thai Prawns en Papillote with Coconut Milk** *(opposite) is another healthy shellfish dish. Coconut milk may be high in saturates, but there is evidence that these don't have the same effect as saturates from animal sources. For 4 as a starter, or 2 as a main course, peel 20 large raw prawns, leaving tails on. Bruise 2 lemon grass stalks, cut in half lengthwise and then into 8 long pieces. Put 2 finely chopped shallots, 1 small red chilli, deseeded and cut into strips, 2 finely chopped garlic cloves, 2.5cm/1in piece of fresh ginger, finely chopped, 4 lime leaves and a generous pinch of turmeric in a pan with 400ml/14fl oz coconut milk. Simmer for 5 minutes. Preheat the oven to 180°C/350°F/Gas 4.*

*Cut out eight 33cm/13inch circles from sheets of baking parchment. Use 2 circles per parcel. Divide the prawns between the 4 parcels. Bring the paper up and shape into a pouch (setting the circles into suitably sized bowls makes it easier). Pour in the coconut milk, making sure each parcel has an even share of all flavourings. Sprinkle 4 tablespoons chopped coriander over the top. Tie up the tops with string. Put on a baking sheet and bake for 10 minutes. Serve the pouches in the bowls, with prawn crackers.*

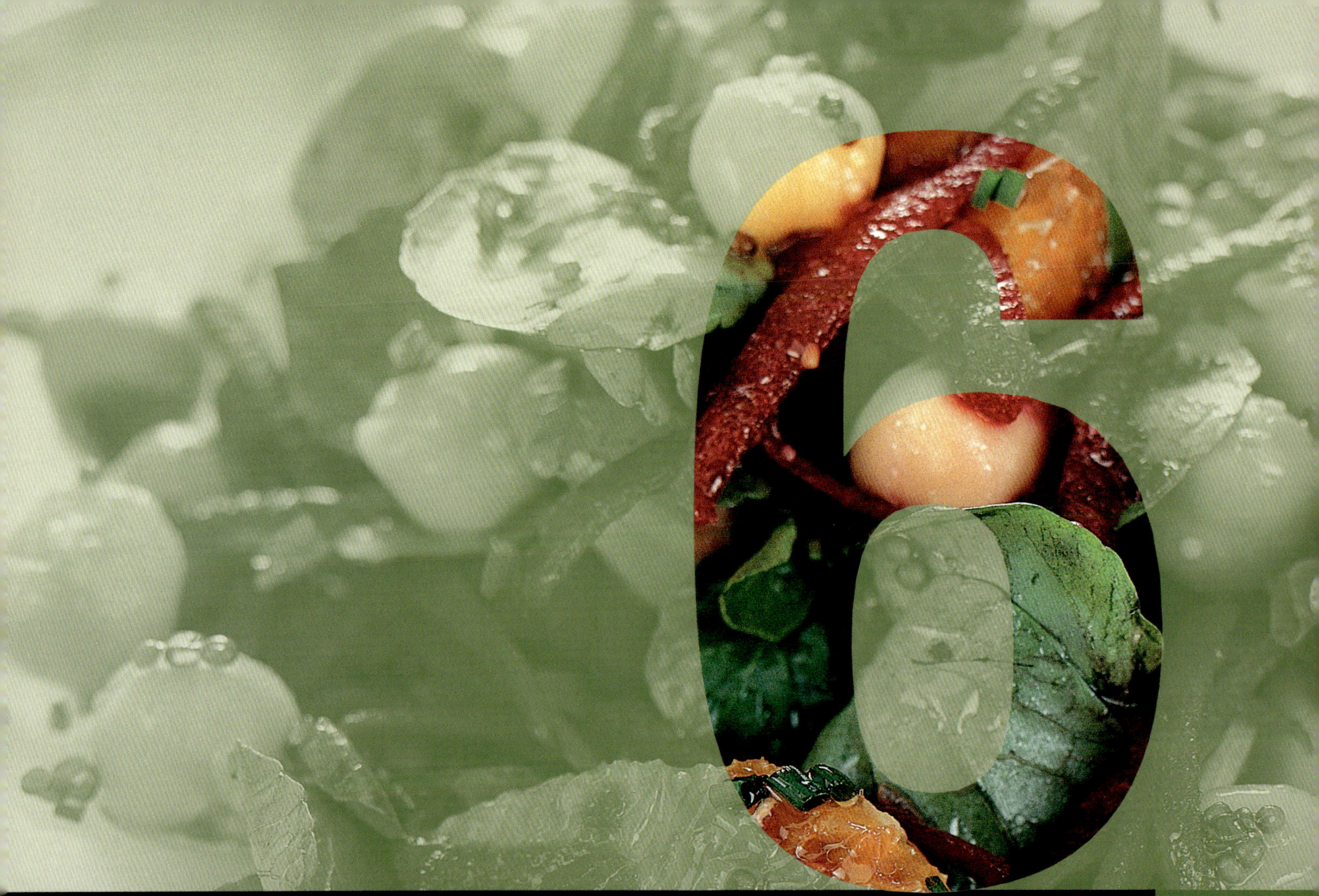


# Spirited Salads and Vegetable Dishes

*Of course, this should be the easiest area in which to ensure healthy eating, but it's amazing how easy it is to lose the many glorious benefits of these intrinsically wholesome ingredients through bad handling or cooking. For maximum benefit, wherever possible prepare vegetables just before they're required, don't leave them soaking in water for hours so their nutrients leach out, and try to cook them as lightly as possible. A good intake of raw vegetables or salads is also recommended all year round - not just in summer!*

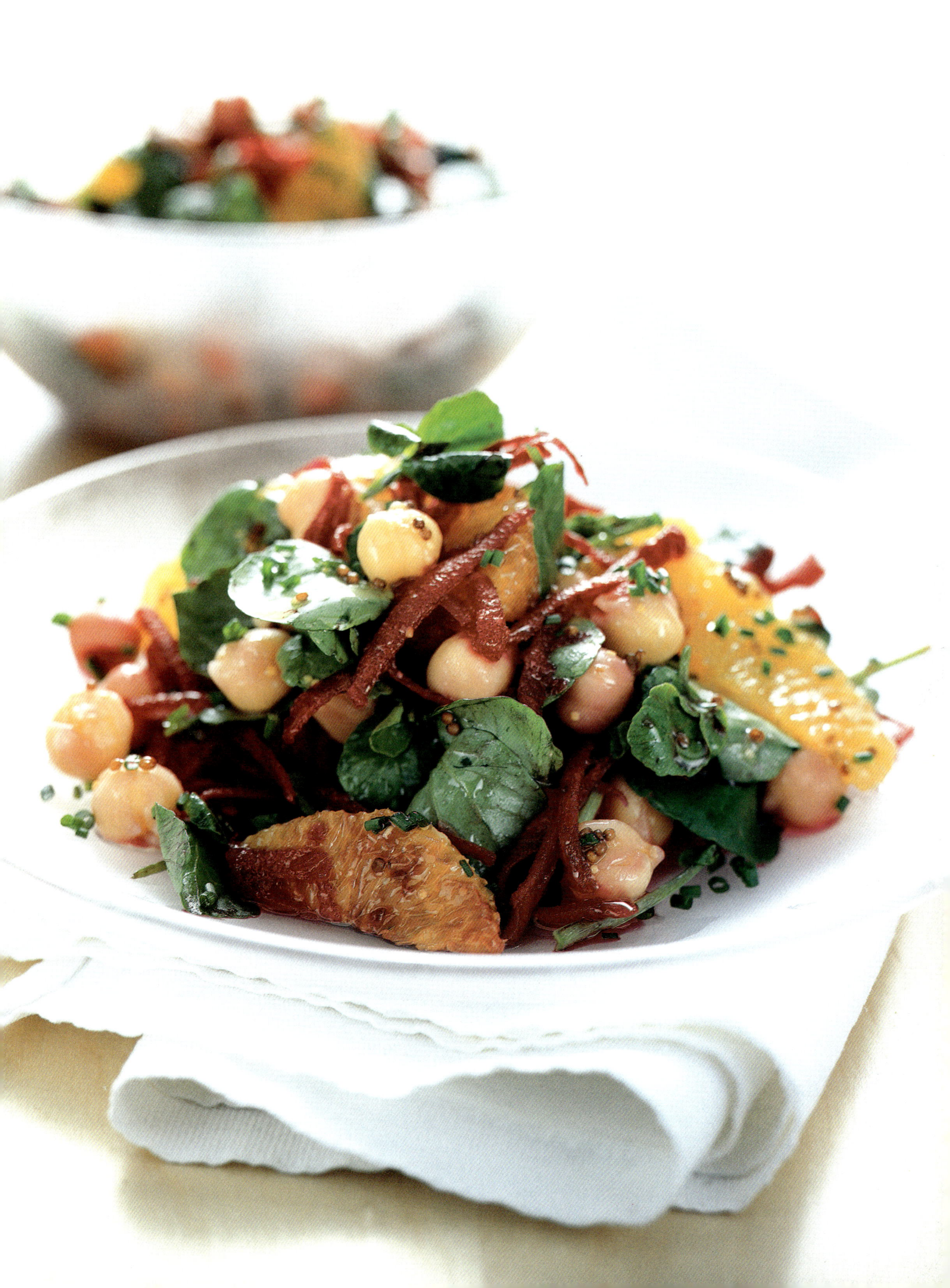

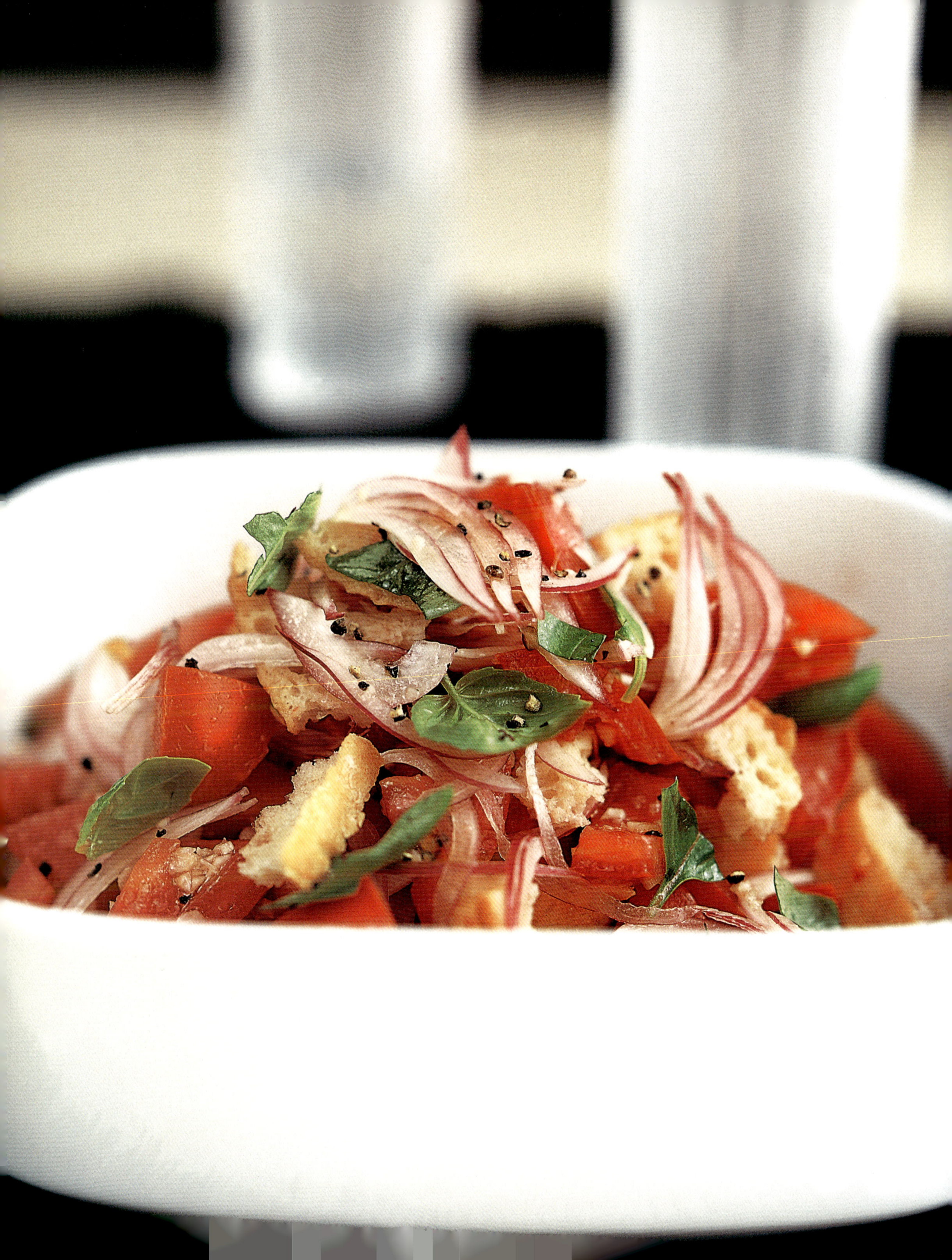

# Beetroot and Chickpea Salad

PER SERVING
217 kcalories
protein 8g
carbohydrate 24g
fat 11g
saturated fat 1g
fibre 6g
added sugar 1g
salt 0.61g

**This tasty and highly nutritious salad will take you halfway towards getting your 'five a day' of fruit and vegetables, and the fact that all but the chickpeas are raw helps to maximize the good that they deliver. Oranges are, of course, a 'superfood' (see page 100), the average fruit containing more than our daily minimum requirement of vitamin C, as well as other highly effective antioxidant phytochemicals. Watercress, too, is full of vitamins and minerals, especially iron. Beetroot is a good source of folate and potassium.**

PREPARATION 20 minutes

2 oranges
410g/14oz can of chickpeas, drained
85g/3oz bag of watercress, roughly chopped
1 raw beetroot, about 300g/10oz, grated

**for the dressing**

1 tsp clear honey
2 tsp wholegrain mustard
1 tbsp lemon juice
3 tbsp olive oil
handful of chopped fresh chives

1 Slice off the tops and bottoms of the oranges, then cut away the peel and pith, leaving just the flesh. Holding each orange over a bowl (to catch the juices), cut down either side of each segment, as close to the skin as possible, to remove.
2 Make the dressing: whisk the honey, mustard, lemon juice, olive oil and reserved orange juice in a bowl. Stir in the chives and season.
3 Toss together the chickpeas, orange segments, watercress and dressing. Stir in the beetroot and serve.

# Panzanella

PER SERVING
183 kcalories
protein 3g
carbohydrate 16g
fat 12g
saturated fat 2g
fibre 2g
added sugar none
salt 0.45g

**This Italian peasant-style salad relies very much on the quality of your ingredients - so pick ripe, juicy, tasty tomatoes and use your best extra-virgin olive oil.**

SERVES 6 as a side salad
PREPARATION 15 minutes
COOKING 20 minutes

1/2 ciabatta loaf
900g/2lb ripe tomatoes
1 red onion, thinly sliced
2 garlic cloves, finely chopped
generous bunch of basil leaves

**for the dressing**

6 tbsp extra-virgin olive oil
3 tbsp red wine vinegar

1 Preheat the oven to 180°C/350°F/Gas 4. Slice the ciabatta fairly thinly, then put the slices on a baking sheet in a single layer. Bake for 10 minutes, then turn the slices over and bake for a further 10 minutes, until the bread is lightly browned and dry. Allow to cool on a wire rack.
2 Cut the tomatoes into small wedges or chop them if they are large. Put them in a large bowl with the onion and garlic. Mix well, then break the bread up into small chunks and add to the tomatoes. Tear the basil leaves into small pieces and add to the bowl. Mix well again.
3 Make the dressing: whisk together the oil, vinegar, salt and pepper. Drizzle the dressing over the salad and mix well. You want the bread to take on the flavours of the basil and oil without getting too soggy, so serve the salad within an hour of making it.

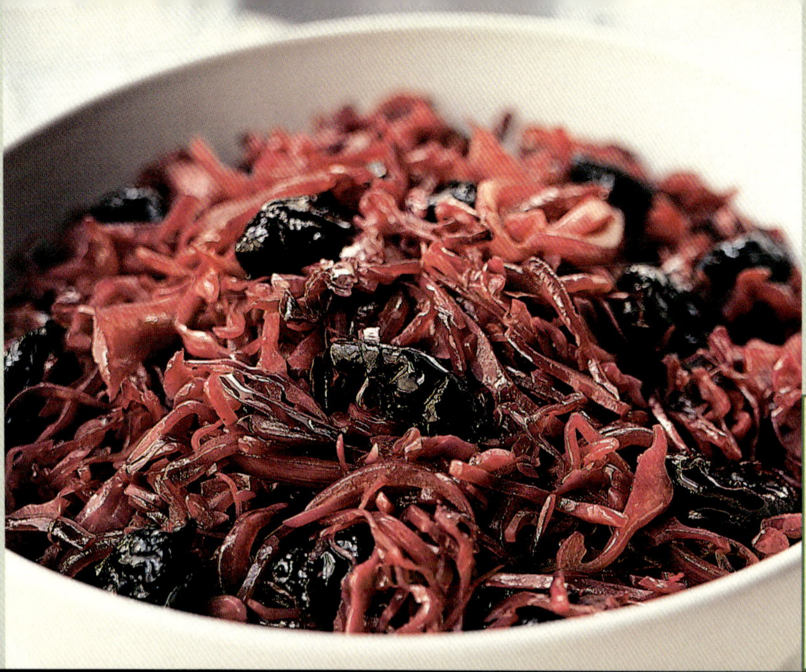

**PER SERVING**
122 kcalories
protein 4g
carbohydrate 2g
fat 11g
saturated fat 2g
fibre 3g
added sugar none
salt 0.47g

## It's a fish, it's a fruit, it's a veg... it's superfood!

### What exactly is a superfood?

*A 'superfood' is the term for a food that not only supplies a wide range of nutrients (without also delivering too many negatives, like saturated fats, etc.) but also contains agents that actively help fight disease.*

### Where are most of the superfoods found?

*Generally, they are plant-based foods, like vegetables, fruits, nuts and grains. It was discovered that these contained a whole range of goodies that were not just necessary for our bodies to function properly, but aided the processes that combat disease. These are called phytochemicals, from 'phyto' meaning plant, and are often present in relatively high quantities, as they tend to be the chemicals responsible for the plant's colour, odour or flavour (hence the emphasis on eating your greens and other deep-coloured vegetables).*

### What are these phytochemicals in superfoods and how do they work?

*They generally fall into a handful of groups. The carotenoids are named after beta-carotene. Responsible for the orange colour in vegetables like carrots, this is converted into vitamin A by the body. Beta-carotene is also a very potent antioxidant, i.e. it helps neutralize damaging 'free radicals' in the body that can cause cell damage and may lead to cancer. Another important carotenoid is lycopene, the red pigment in tomatoes, which seems to be enormously powerful in its antioxidant effect, reducing the risk of some cancers, notably of the prostate, lungs and stomach.*

*The bioflavonoids are mostly found in fruit, notably citrus fruits, berries, cherries and grapes. Potent antioxidants, each particular flavonoid seems to help fight a particular range of conditions, particularly cancers.*

*The glucinolates are prevalent in the cabbage family and other greens. Those in broccoli, for example, stimulate our natural defences and those in Brussels sprouts combat growth of pre-cancerous cells.*

*The organosulphides are mostly found in the onion family, like onions, garlic and leeks. They reinforce the immune system and combat heart disease and cancers, especially of the digestive system.*

*Phyto-oestrogens mimic the female hormone, protecting against osteoporosis, heart disease and breast and womb cancer. They also alleviate a range of female problems, especially menopause-related. Sources are pulses, especially soya beans, and some grains, seeds and berries, notably flax seeds (linseeds).*

### Are there any superfoods that are not from plants?

*Yes, oily fish (like salmon, tuna, mackerel, herring and sardines) that are rich in omega-3 oils* *(see page 76).*

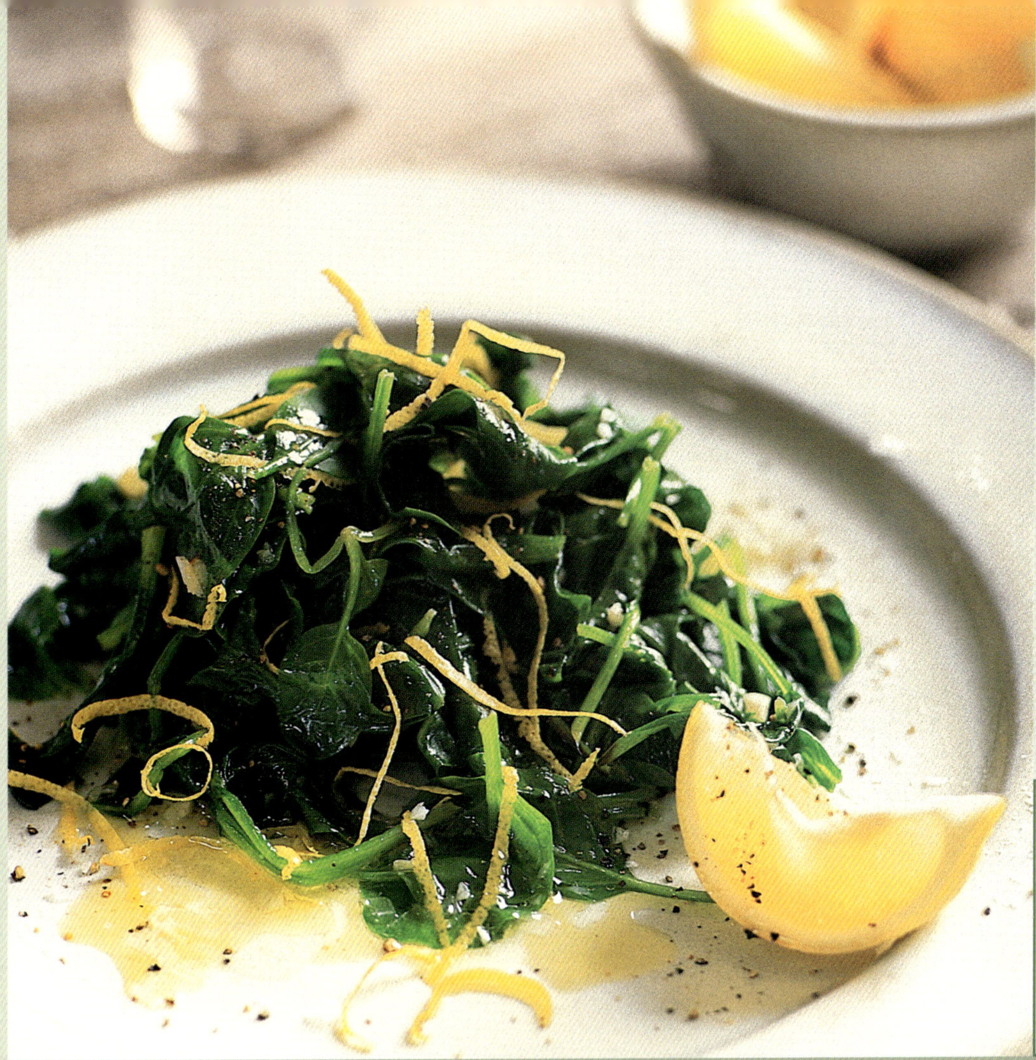

**PER PANCAKE**
**248 kcalories**
**protein 10g**
**carbohydrate 29g**
**fat 11g**
**saturated fat 6g**
**fibre 1g**
**added sugar 10g**
**salt 0.24g**

**The superfood message is not unlike the 'five-a-day' dictum: build a wide range of different fruits, seeds, grains and vegetables into your diet to benefit from this fantastic armoury of wonderful 'natural medicines' ▼**

## Garlic Lemon Spinach

*(above) is delicious and healthy as a course served between courses, or as a quick snack. It must be prepared and eaten straight away so the lemon has no time to blacken the tender young spinach leaves.*

*Heat 4 tablespoons olive oil in a wok or large frying pan, then fry 3 finely chopped garlic cloves, until just sizzling, but not browned. Add half of 500g/1lb 2oz young spinach leaves and stir until just wilted; transfer to a dish and keep warm while you cook the remaining spinach. Toss all the spinach with the juice and grated zest of $^1/_2$ lemon and season with sea salt and black pepper. Divide between 4 serving plates and serve immediately with lemon wedges.*

## Red Cabbage with Prunes

*(opposite) goes well with duck, or roast pork or turkey. Heat 2 tablespoons olive oil in a large wide pan, then add 1 sliced red onion and cook for a few minutes to soften. Add 800g/1lb 12oz shredded red cabbage and cook, stirring, over a moderate heat for 5–7 minutes. Stir in 250g/9oz halved pitted prunes, the juice of 1 large orange, 2 tablespoons balsamic vinegar and a teaspoon of salt.*

*Cover the pan with a tight-fitting lid and simmer gently for 30 minutes, stirring occasionally, until the cabbage is cooked but still has a bit of bite. Add a little water to the pan if the cabbage becomes too dry.*

# Tian of Root Vegetables

**PER SERVING**
**101 kcalories**
**protein 2g**
**carbohydrate 15g**
**fat 4g**
**saturated fat 1g**
**fibre 3g**
**added sugar trace**
**salt 0.35g**

**The orange-fleshed sweet potato is rich in antioxidant, cancer-fighting beta-carotene, making it a 'superfood' (see page 100); unfortunately the paler-fleshed varieties don't have this advantage.**

PREPARATION 35 minutes
COOKING about 1 hour

2 small sweet potatoes (orange-fleshed if you can get them)
2 medium potatoes
1 small celeriac, about 300g/10oz
2 small parsnips
4 tbsp olive oil, plus more for greasing
2–3 tbsp chopped fresh parsley, plus more to garnish

1 Preheat the oven to 200°C/400°F/Gas 6. Peel all the vegetables, then thinly slice with a mandolin or in a food processor (or slice them very thinly by hand).
2 Blanch the vegetable slices in a pan of boiling salted water for 3–5 minutes (no longer or they will break up). Drain, reserving some of the cooking liquid, and refresh under cold running water.
3 Oil two 25cm/10in shallow ovenproof dishes. Layer the vegetables randomly; between each layer, sprinkle some parsley, salt and pepper, and drizzle with oil. Pour in just enough liquid to cover the first layer of vegetables. Cover loosely with a double sheet of oiled greaseproof paper.
4 Bake for 30 minutes, uncover and cook for 30 minutes more until tender and golden.
5 Garnish with parsley to serve.

# New Vegetables à la Grecque

**PER SERVING**
**322 kcalories**
**protein 11g**
**carbohydrate 36g**
**fat 16g**
**saturated fat 2g**
**fibre 12g**
**added sugar none**
**salt 0.67g**

**This is great as an accompaniment or starter. You could use mangetout or sugar snap peas instead of broad beans.**

PREPARATION 15 minutes
COOKING 25 minutes

5 tbsp olive oil
1 large garlic clove, crushed
3 baby aubergines or 1 small aubergine (about 85g/3oz), chopped into small dice
1 red (or ordinary) onion, thinly sliced
1 large tomato, skinned and chopped
3 tbsp sun-dried tomato paste
2 tbsp red wine vinegar
450g/1lb baby new potatoes, scrubbed and halved
350g/12oz baby carrots, trimmed and halved
450g/1lb broad beans, shelled
100g/4oz young asparagus spears
**to serve**
30g/1oz black olives
1 tbsp capers
fresh flat-leaf parsley leaves

1 Heat the olive oil in a frying pan, then add the garlic, aubergine and onion, and cook over a moderate heat until very soft (about 10 minutes).
2 Transfer the mixture to a very large bowl and stir in the chopped tomato and sun-dried tomato paste. Add the red wine vinegar and season to taste with salt and pepper.
3 Cook the potatoes and carrots in a pan of lightly salted boiling water for about 15 minutes until tender, then drain well. Meanwhile, steam the broad beans and asparagus for about 5 minutes until just tender.
4 While still hot, tip the vegetables into the aubergine mixture. Stir well to coat and leave to cool for about 5 minutes before serving, so they have a chance to absorb the flavours of the sauce.
5 Serve sprinkled with black olives, capers and parsley leaves.

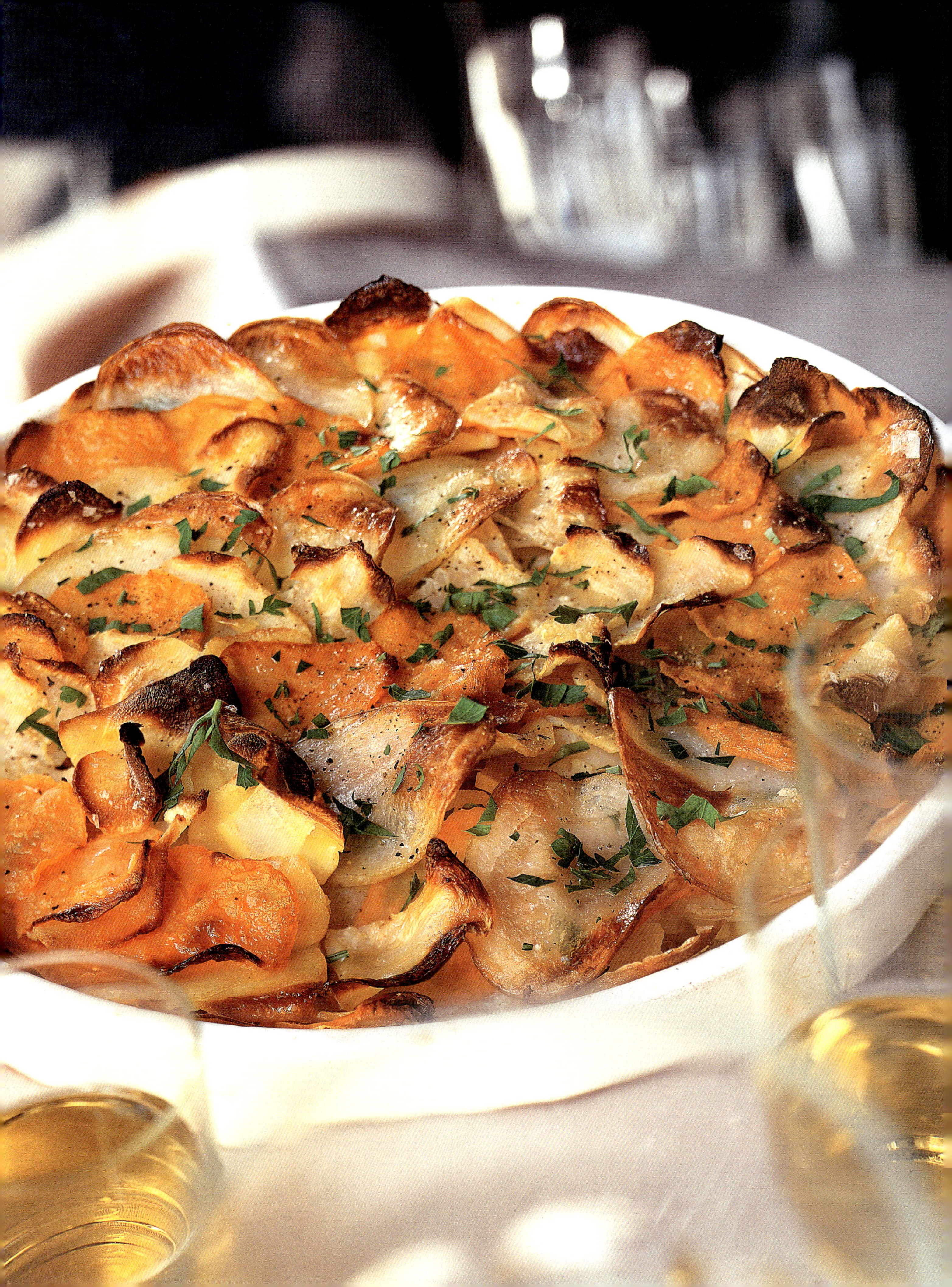

# Roasted Vegetable Rice

**PREPARATION** 15 minutes
**COOKING** 25 minutes

4 courgettes, cut into chunks
2 yellow peppers, deseeded and cut into chunks
1 large onion, cut into wedges
3 tbsp olive oil
6 tomatoes, each cut into 6 wedges
3 garlic cloves, finely chopped
½ tsp chilli flakes or powder
½ tsp ground turmeric
350g/12oz long-grain rice
100g/4oz Cheddar cheese, cut into cubes

1 Preheat the oven to 220°C/425°F/Gas 7. Put the courgettes, peppers and onion in a roasting tin. Drizzle over the olive oil and season. Roast for 15 minutes, then add the tomatoes and sprinkle with garlic and chilli. Cook for 10 minutes more, until softened but not mushy.
2 Meanwhile, bring a kettleful of water to the boil, pour the water into a large pan and bring back to the boil. Stir in the turmeric, then tip in the rice and cook for 10–12 minutes until tender. Drain, return to the pan and stir in the cheese.
3 Pile the rice on to serving plates, spoon over the vegetables and drizzle with some of the juices.

**VARIATIONS**

Instead of adding turmeric and Cheddar to the rice, sprinkle the vegetables with Parmesan. Alternatively, try placing 8 streaky bacon rashers over the vegetables while roasting and cook until crisp, then serve them on top.

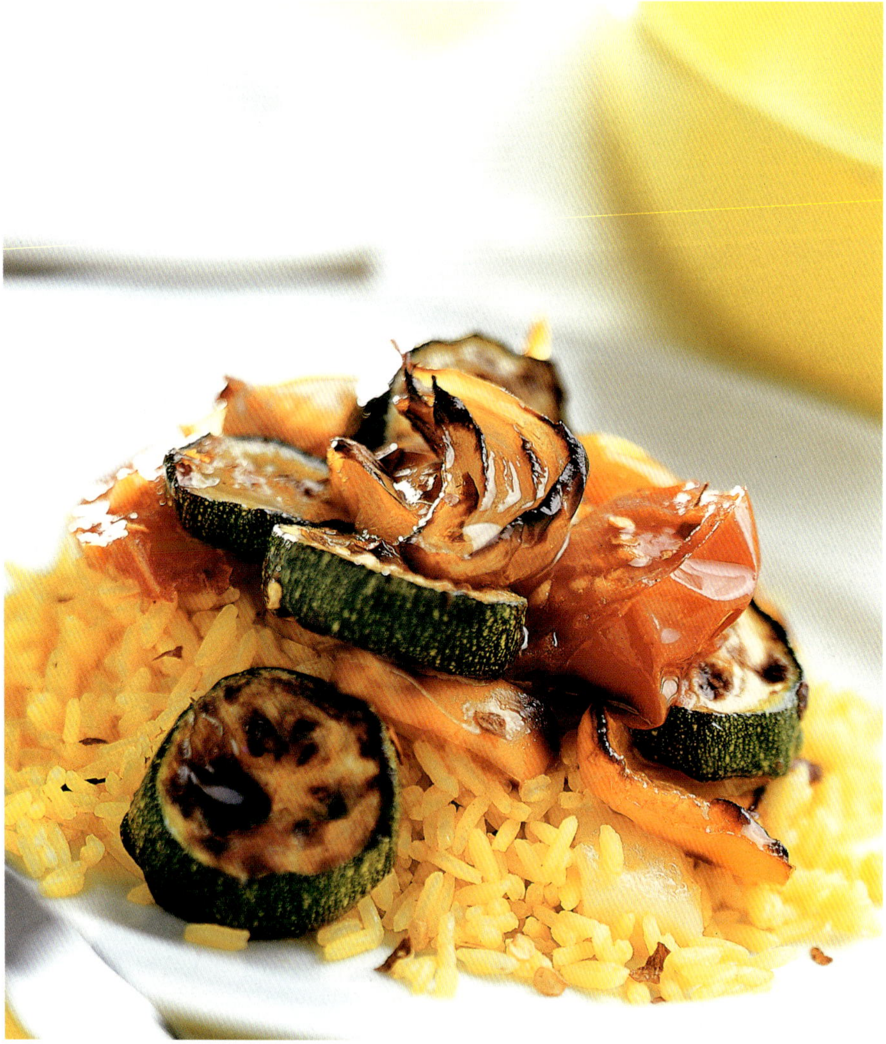

**PER SERVING**
**577 kcalories**
**protein 17g**
**carbohydrate 91g**
**fat 19g**
**saturated fat 7g**
**fibre 4g**
**added sugar none**
**salt 0.75g**

# Seven-vegetable Couscous

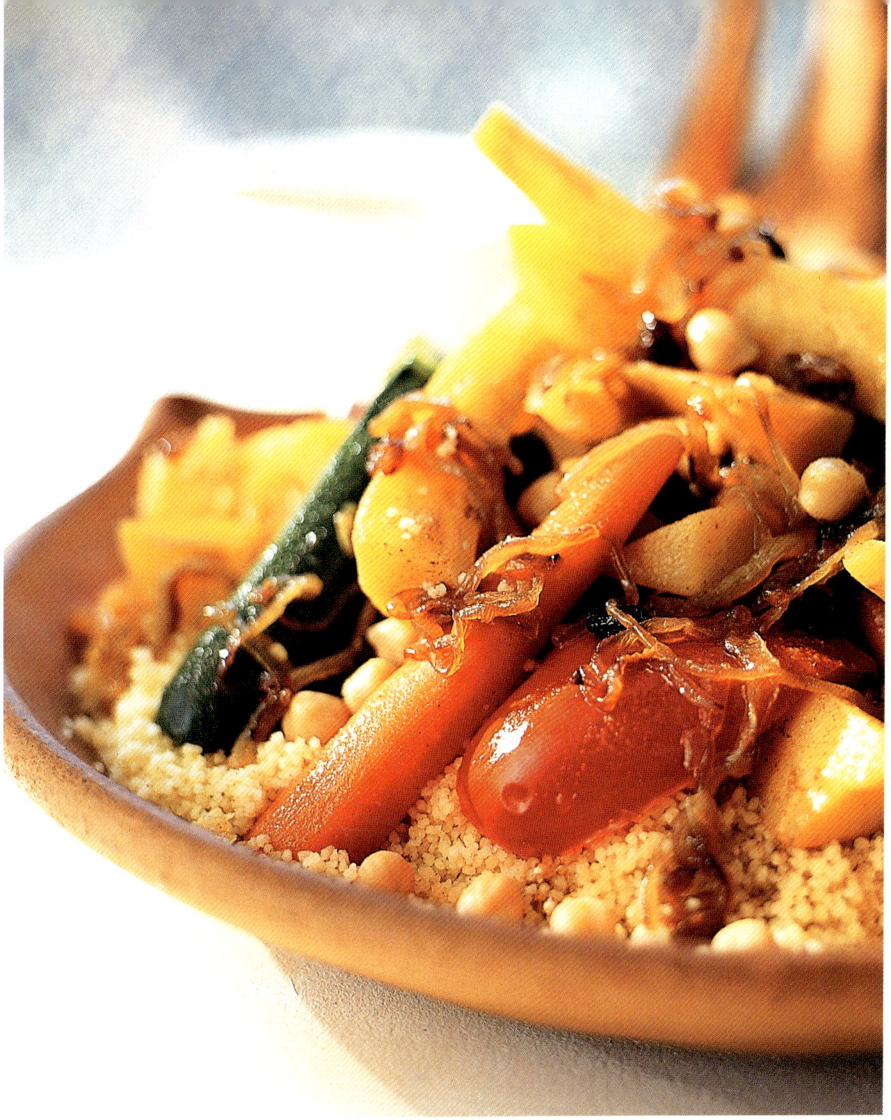

1.2 litres/2 pints good vegetable stock
½ tsp ground paprika, plus more to serve
½ tsp ground cinnamon, plus more to serve
½ tsp ground cumin, plus more to serve
pinch of cayenne pepper, plus more to serve
pinch of ground ginger, plus more to serve
2 good pinches of saffron threads
2 medium potatoes
4 small turnips
4 parsnips
1 swede
6 small carrots
500g/1lb 2oz couscous
500ml/18fl oz boiling water
3 small courgettes
2 red peppers, quartered and deseeded

**to serve**

400g/14 oz can of chickpeas, drained
1 Spanish onion, thinly sliced
30g/1oz butter
2 tbsp clear honey
harissa
a little olive oil or butter
6 tbsp raisins, plumped up in water

PER SERVING
**389 kcalories**
**protein 11g**
**carbohydrate 73g**
**fat 8g**
**saturated fat 2g**
**fibre 9g**
**added sugar 3g**
**salt 1.18g**

SERVES
8 (easily halved)
PREPARATION
15 minutes
COOKING
25 minutes

**Harissa is a fiery and versatile Moroccan condiment, now available in many better supermarkets. This hot paste is made of dried chilli peppers, garlic, coriander, salt and cumin. Stir a little into stews and couscous or use a thinner version as a dressing for salads.**

1 Put the stock in the base of a large pan which has a tight-fitting steamer. Add the paprika, cinnamon, cumin, cayenne, ginger and saffron and bring to a simmer over a moderate heat.
2 Peel all the root vegetables. Cut each potato into 6 wedges. Cut the turnips and swede into similar wedges. Cut the parsnips lengthwise into quarters or halves. Add the potatoes, turnips, parsnips and swede to the stock. Simmer, covered, for 15 minutes.
3 Meanwhile, put the couscous in a bowl and pour over the boiling water. Let stand for 15 minutes.
4 Add the carrots, courgettes and peppers to the stock. Cover and cook for 20 minutes more.
5 Line the steamer with wet muslin. Add the couscous and place on top of the stew to warm.
6 Heat the chickpeas in a little stock and keep warm. Fry the onion in butter and honey until soft; keep warm.
7 Tip the couscous into a large bowl and separate with a fork. Work in a little oil or butter, a pinch or two of salt, paprika, cinnamon, cumin, cayenne and ginger and fork through. Ladle in a little stock, flavoured with harissa, to moisten.
8 Pile the couscous on to a large serving plate, making a well in the middle. Arrange the drained veg around the sides and on top of the couscous. Scatter over the chickpeas, raisins and onion. Serve with a bowl of the stock flavoured with a teaspoon of harissa.

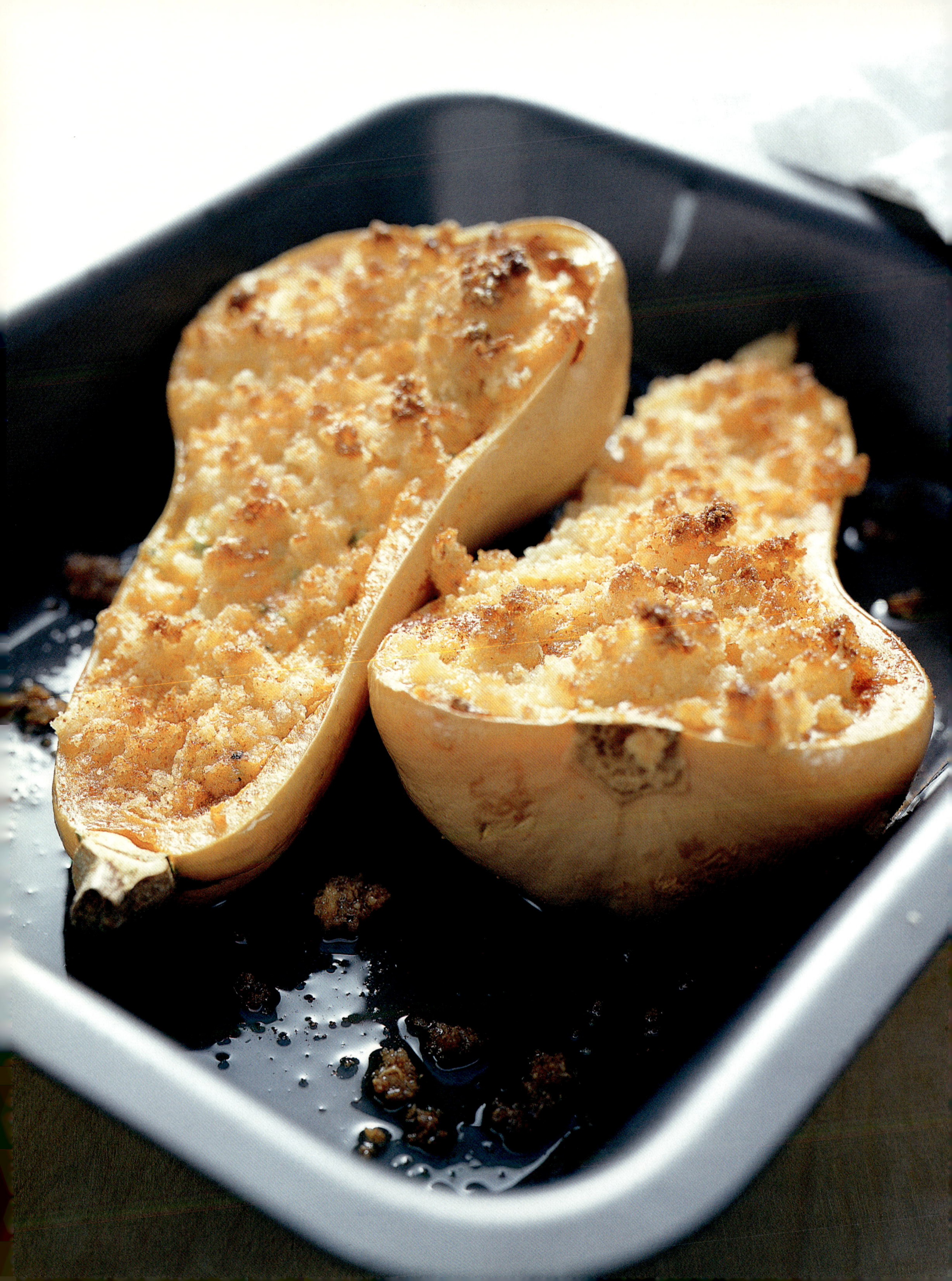

# Baked Buttery Squash

PER SERVING
**271 kcalories**
**protein 13g**
**carbohydrate 35g**
**fat 10g**
**saturated fat 6g**
**fibre 5g**
**added sugar none**
**salt 0.78g**

**Butternut squash, being orange-fleshed, is rich in protective carotenoids, as well as the antioxidant vitamins C and E.**

SERVES 2
PREPARATION 10 minutes
COOKING about 1 hour

1 butternut squash, about 675g/1½lb
½ tsp paprika
3 tbsp snipped fresh chives
3 tbsp low-fat crème fraîche
1 thick slice of white bread, crust removed, crumbled into breadcrumbs
generous knob of butter, melted
30g/1oz grated Parmesan cheese

1 Preheat the oven to 200°C/400°F/Gas 6. Halve the squash lengthwise, then scoop out the seeds and fibres. Season well and put in a roasting tin half full of water. Cover with foil and bake for about 40 minutes until the squash is tender, but not collapsing.
2 Drain off the water. Transfer the squash to a board and leave until cool enough to handle, then scrape the flesh into a bowl, leaving a thin border of flesh on the skin.
3 Mix the paprika, chives and crème fraîche into the flesh and season. Pile the mixture into the squash shells. Mix the breadcrumbs with the butter and Parmesan and sprinkle on top.
4 Bake for 15 minutes until lightly browned.

# Spiced Vegetable Pancake Stack

PER SERVING
**405 kcalories**
**protein 13g**
**carbohydrate 40g**
**fat 22g**
**saturated fat 4g**
**fibre 5g**
**added sugar none**
**salt 0.85g**

PREPARATION 30 minutes
COOKING 30 minutes

handful of chopped fresh coriander
1 quantity of pancake batter (page 17)
2 tbsp sunflower oil
1 small onion, finely chopped
500g/1lb 2oz bag of prepared mixed vegetables (carrots, broccoli and cauliflower)
1 tsp ground cumin
2 tsp ground coriander
½ tsp turmeric
two 300g/10½ oz tubs of fresh tomato sauce
lime or lemon wedges, to serve

1 Stir half the chopped coriander into the batter and cook the pancakes as in the master recipe. Cover with foil and set aside. Preheat the oven to 180°C/350°F/Gas 4.
2 Heat the oil in a frying pan and fry the onion for 5 minutes until golden. Add the vegetables and cook for a further 5 minutes, then add the spices and cook for a minute. Add the tomato sauce, bring to the boil, then cover and simmer for 10 minutes until the vegetables are tender. Stir in the remaining coriander.
3 Layer the vegetables and pancakes in an ovenproof dish, finishing with a pancake. Bake for 10 minutes until hot.
4 Cut into 4 wedges and serve with the lime or lemon wedges.

# Thai Vegetable Curry

**Using interesting, widely available vegetables like marrow or sweet potato as the basis for a curry is a cheap and lively way to meet nutritional needs.**

SERVES 6
PREPARATION 15 minutes
COOKING 20 minutes

1 tbsp vegetable oil
1 large onion, diced
500g/1 lb 2oz sweet potatoes, cubed
300g/10oz squash or marrow, cubed
250g/9oz flat green beans
2 tomatoes, diced
two 400g/14oz cans of coconut milk
2 tsp Thai red curry paste
juice of 1 large lime
2 tbsp soy sauce
handful of fresh basil or coriander
boiled rice, to serve

1 Heat the oil in a large pan and cook the onion, sweet potato and squash for 5 minutes until beginning to soften. Cut the beans into 5cm/2in lengths, then add these and the tomatoes and cook for a further 2–3 minutes, until the tomatoes begin to soften.
2 Add the coconut milk and curry paste and bring to the boil. Cook the mixture for 10–12 minutes until the vegetables are tender. Add the lime juice, soy sauce and fresh basil or coriander. Adjust the seasoning.
3 Serve the curry with plain boiled rice.

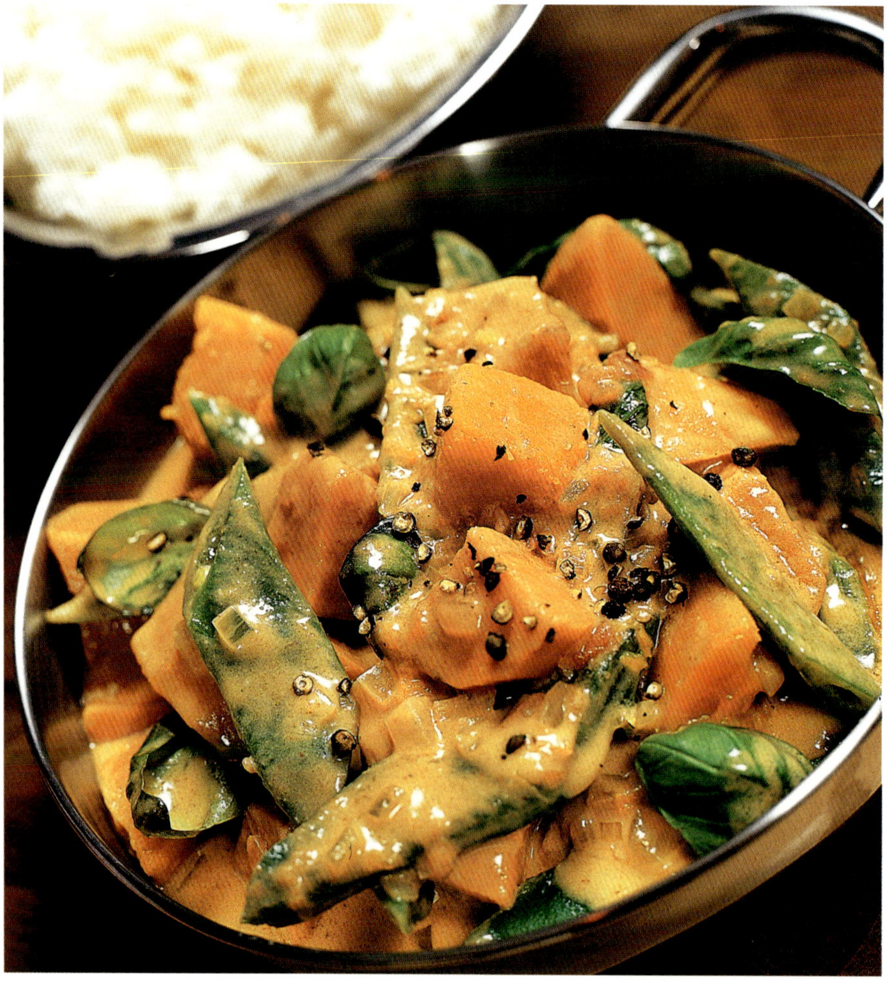

PER SERVING
**354 kcalories**
**protein 5g**
**carbohydrate 31g**
**fat 24g**
**saturated fat 19**
**fibre 4g**
**added sugar none**
**salt 1.44g**

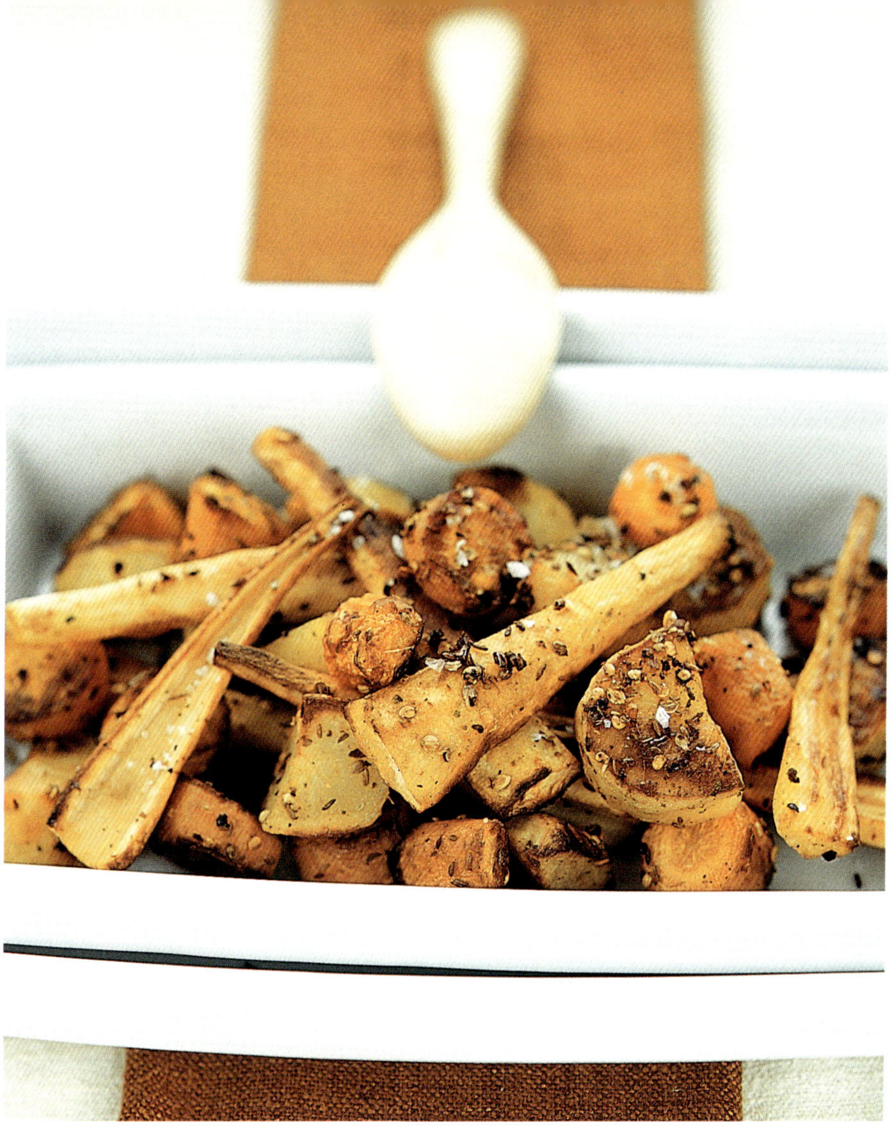

| PER SERVING |
| --- |
| 266 kcalories |
| protein 5g |
| carbohydrate 39g |
| fat 11g |
| saturated fat 3g |
| fibre 7g |
| added sugar none |
| salt 0.53g |

# Roasted Roots with Indian Spices

**To ensure your roast vegetables get a lovely crisp finish, add salt after cooking rather than before – if you sprinkle it over before roasting the salt draws out the vegetables' moisture, which means they'll steam rather than roast.**

SERVES 6
PREPARATION 10 minutes
COOKING 1 hour

2 tsp cumin seeds
2 tsp coriander seeds
2 tsp mixed peppercorns
1 tsp crushed dried chillies
3 tbsp olive oil
30g/1oz butter, melted
675g/1½lb floury potatoes, such as Maris Piper or Cara
450g/1lb carrots
450g/1lb parsnips
sea salt flakes

1 Preheat the oven to 200°C/400°F/Gas 6. Put the cumin, coriander, peppercorns and chillies in mortar and grind with the pestle until they are coarsely ground (if you don't have a pestle and mortar, put the spices in a cup or bowl and grind with the end of a rolling pin). Mix the ground spices with the oil and butter.
2 Peel the potatoes, carrots and parsnips and cut into chunks, or halve lengthwise. Put in a roasting tin large enough to take them in a single layer. Pour the spice mixture over the vegetables and toss everything together so the vegetables are well coated.
3 Roast for about 1 hour until golden and crisp, turning the vegetables a couple of times during cooking so they brown evenly. Sprinkle with sea salt and serve.

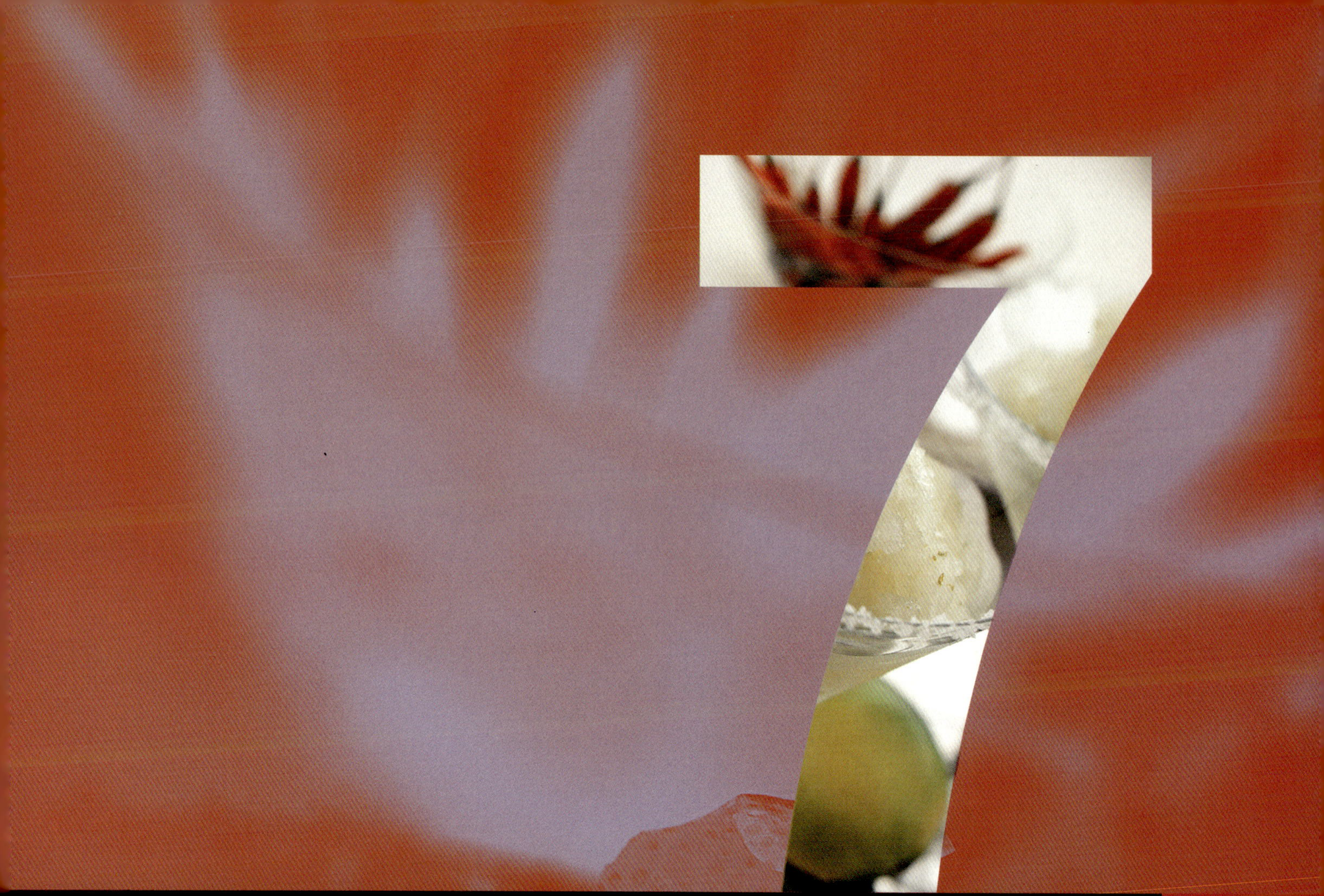

# Prudent Puds

*By its very nature, the sweet course is often seen by healthy eaters as either a 'no-no' or a minefield, but this need not be the case. For a start it is an excellent opportunity to work more fruit, seeds, nuts and grains into your diet. Also, if you are sensible about quantities, you can add luxurious treats like cream and chocolate to such ingredients without compromising the good effects of the whole dish.*

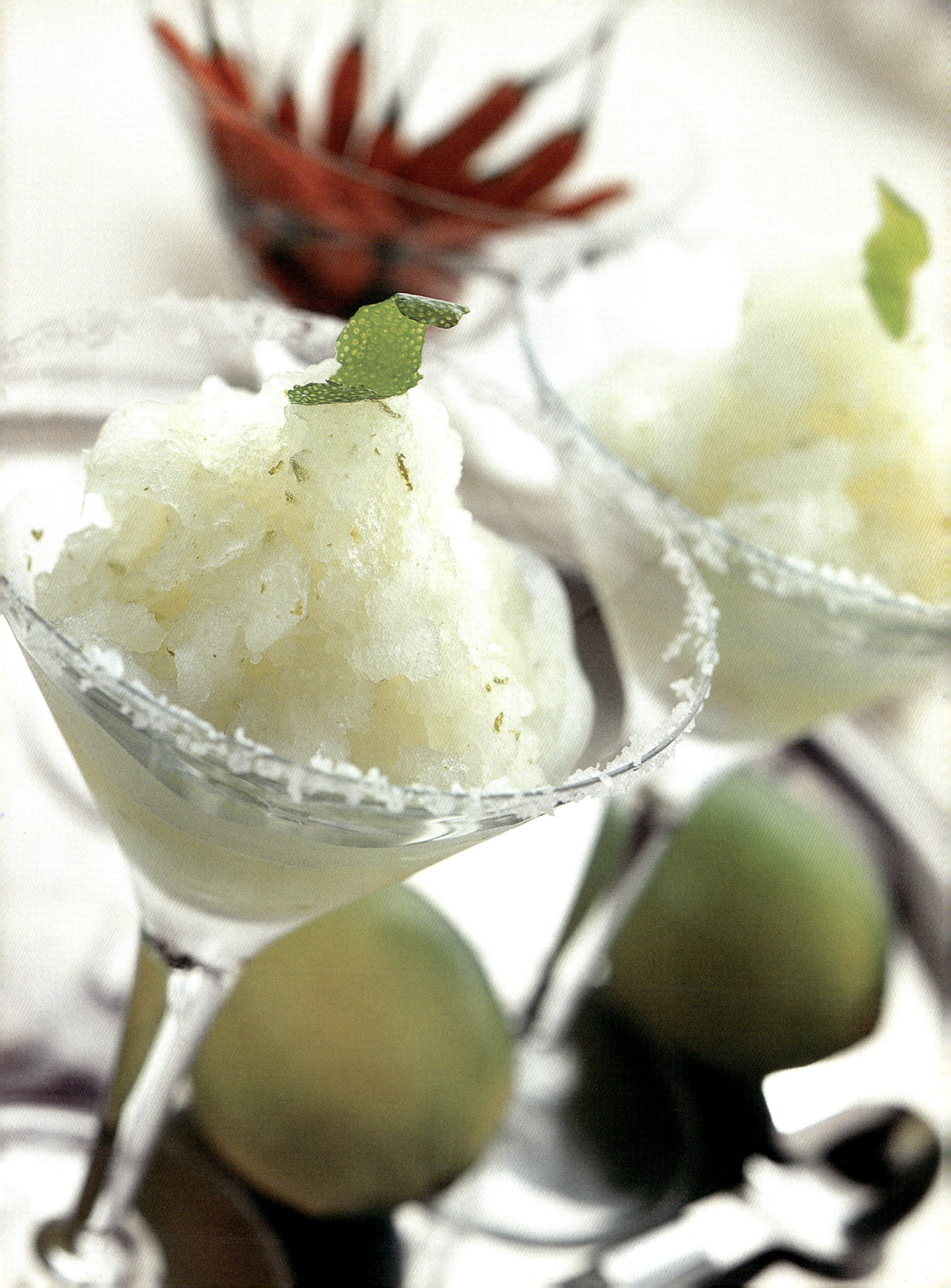

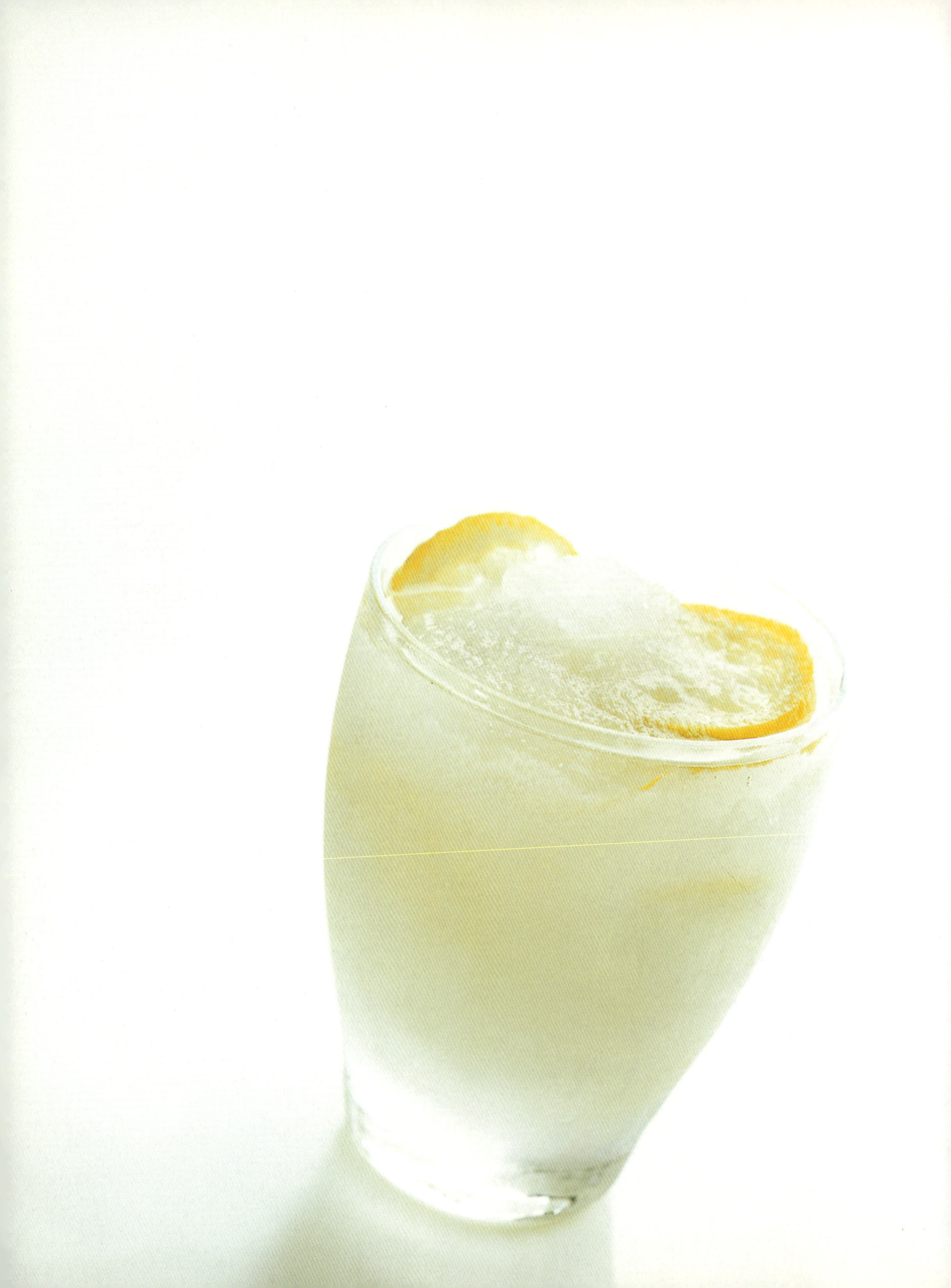

# Margarita Chilli Sorbet

PER SERVING
181 kcalories
protein trace
carbohydrate 44g
fat trace
saturated fat none
fibre none
added sugar 44g
salt 0.02g

**This may sounds like an extraordinary combination, but it tastes quite delicious. Use a medium-sized chilli such as a serrano, or even two if you really want to live on the edge. Remember how healthy chillies are - packed full of vitamin C and other potent antioxidants.**

SERVES 6
PREPARATION 5 minutes
COOKING/FREEZING 4 hours

1 medium-hot fresh red chilli
4 limes
250g/9oz caster sugar
4 tbsp Tequila

1 Trim the stalk from the chilli, leaving the end intact. Using a sharp knife, slash down the length of the chilli skin, starting below the stalk, without disturbing the seeds.
2 Grate the zest from 2 of the limes and cut some of the rind from the others into long strips; reserve the strips for decoration. Squeeze the juice from all 4 limes.
3 Tip the sugar into a pan and pour in 850ml/$1^1/_2$ pints of water. Stir over a gentle heat until the sugar has dissolved. Drop in the chilli and grated zest, then bring to the boil. Simmer for 2 minutes, then remove from the heat, cover and leave until cold (about 1 hour).
4 Take the chilli out of the syrup and discard. Stir in the lime juice and Tequila. Pour into an ice-cream machine and churn for 30–40 minutes until almost frozen, or see below. Transfer to a covered rigid plastic container. Freeze for 2 hours until solid.
5 Before serving, allow to soften in the fridge for 15–30 minutes. Spoon into glasses and decorate with twists of lime rind. For an authentic look, rub the rims of the glasses with half a lime, then dip in coarse sea salt.

# Gin and Tonic Granita

PER SERVING
177 kcalories
protein trace
carbohydrate 25g
fat trace
saturated fat none
fibre none
added sugar 24g
salt 0.02g

**The gin prevents the mixture from freezing solidly, which gives it that traditional icy granita texture.**

PREPARATION 10 minutes
COOKING 5 minutes, plus 30 minutes' cooling and overnight freezing

300ml/$^1/_2$ pint tonic water
30g/1oz caster sugar
150ml/$^1/_4$ pint gin
1 small lemon, thinly sliced

1 Put the tonic water and sugar in a pan and bring to the boil, stirring until the sugar dissolves. Remove from the heat and allow to cool for about 30 minutes.
2 Stir in the gin, then spoon the mixture into a rigid container and freeze for 2–3 hours until semi-frozen. Stir to distribute the ice crystals evenly through the mixture, then return to the freezer. Leave overnight until the granita is firm but crumbles when a spoon is scraped across the surface.
3 Spoon the mixture into 4 small tumblers, pushing lemon slices into the mixture as you go. Serve immediately or freeze until needed.

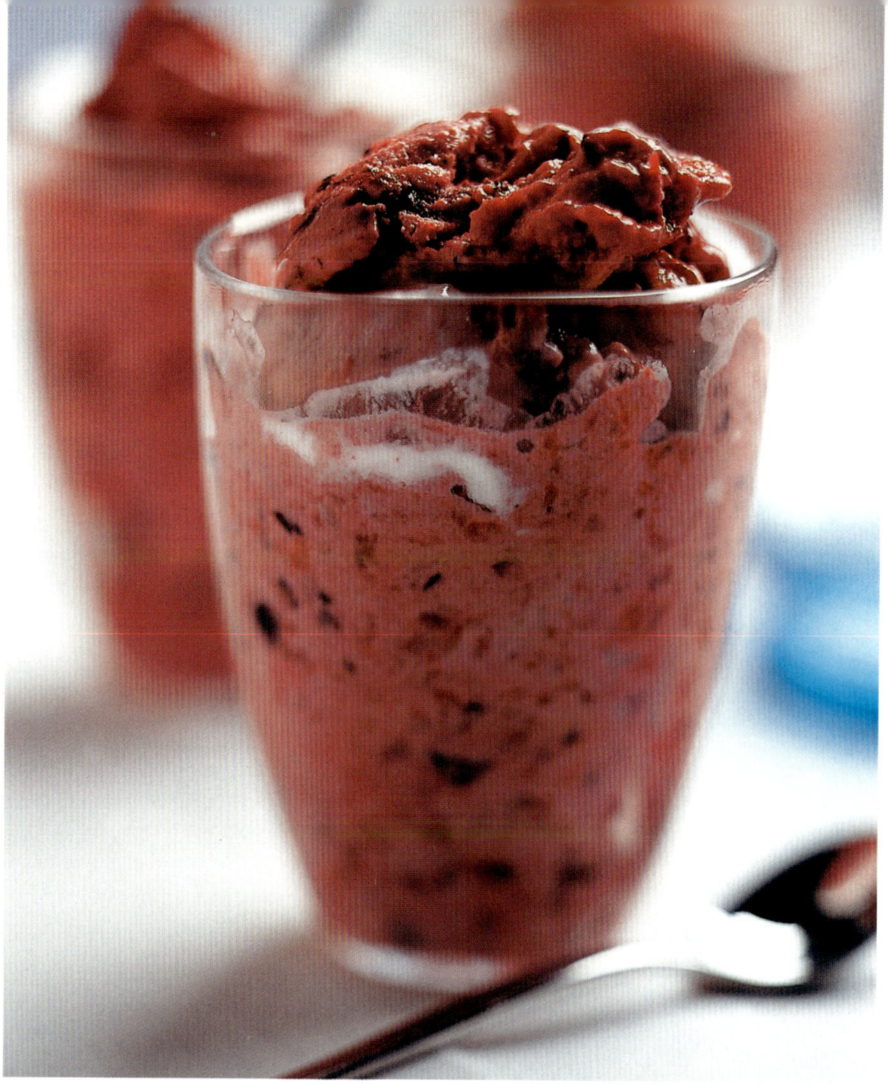

PER SERVING
184 kcalories
protein 8g
carbohydrate 18g
fat 9g
saturated fat 6g
fibre 3g
added sugar 7g
salt 0.2g

# Summer Fruits Ice Yoghurt

PREPARATION about 10 minutes

500g/1lb 2oz bag of frozen mixed summer fruits
two 200g/7oz tubs of Greek-style yoghurt
100ml/3½fl oz (about 7 tbsp) fresh orange juice
1 tbsp icing sugar

VARIATION

You can, of course, use lemon or lime juice for a sharper flavour.

1 Put the frozen fruits, yoghurt, orange juice and icing sugar in a food processor. Process until blended, but make sure the fruit still retains some texture. You may need to scrape the mixture down the sides of the processor once or twice between bursts so that everything is incorporated. The mixture will quickly look like frozen yoghurt.

2 Spoon the mixture into chunky glasses to serve.

# Frozen Redcurrant and Ginger Crush

PER SERVING
226 kcalories
protein 9g
carbohydrate 24g
fat 11g
saturated fat 7g
fibre 2g
added sugar 19g
salt 0.27g

**To give a ginger flavour but not an overpowering one, you can use a little syrup from a jar of stem ginger. If you don't have any stem ginger, add a small very finely chopped piece of crystallized ginger instead.**

PREPARATION 5 minutes, plus 2 hours' freezing

225g/8oz redcurrants, destalked
1 tbsp syrup from a jar of stem ginger
4 tbsp icing sugar
500ml/18fl oz tub of Greek-style yoghurt

1 Reserve a few of the redcurrants for decoration, then put the rest in a food processor with the ginger syrup and icing sugar. Switch on the machine, pour in the yoghurt and process until just blended.
2 Transfer the mixture to a rigid plastic container and cover. Freeze for 2 hours until semi-frozen, but still soft enough to scoop.
3 Scoop the dessert into serving bowls and decorate with reserved redcurrants.

VARIATION
It's just as easy to use frozen redcurrants in this recipe. There's no need to defrost them, so the dessert will only need to be frozen for 1–1½ hours.

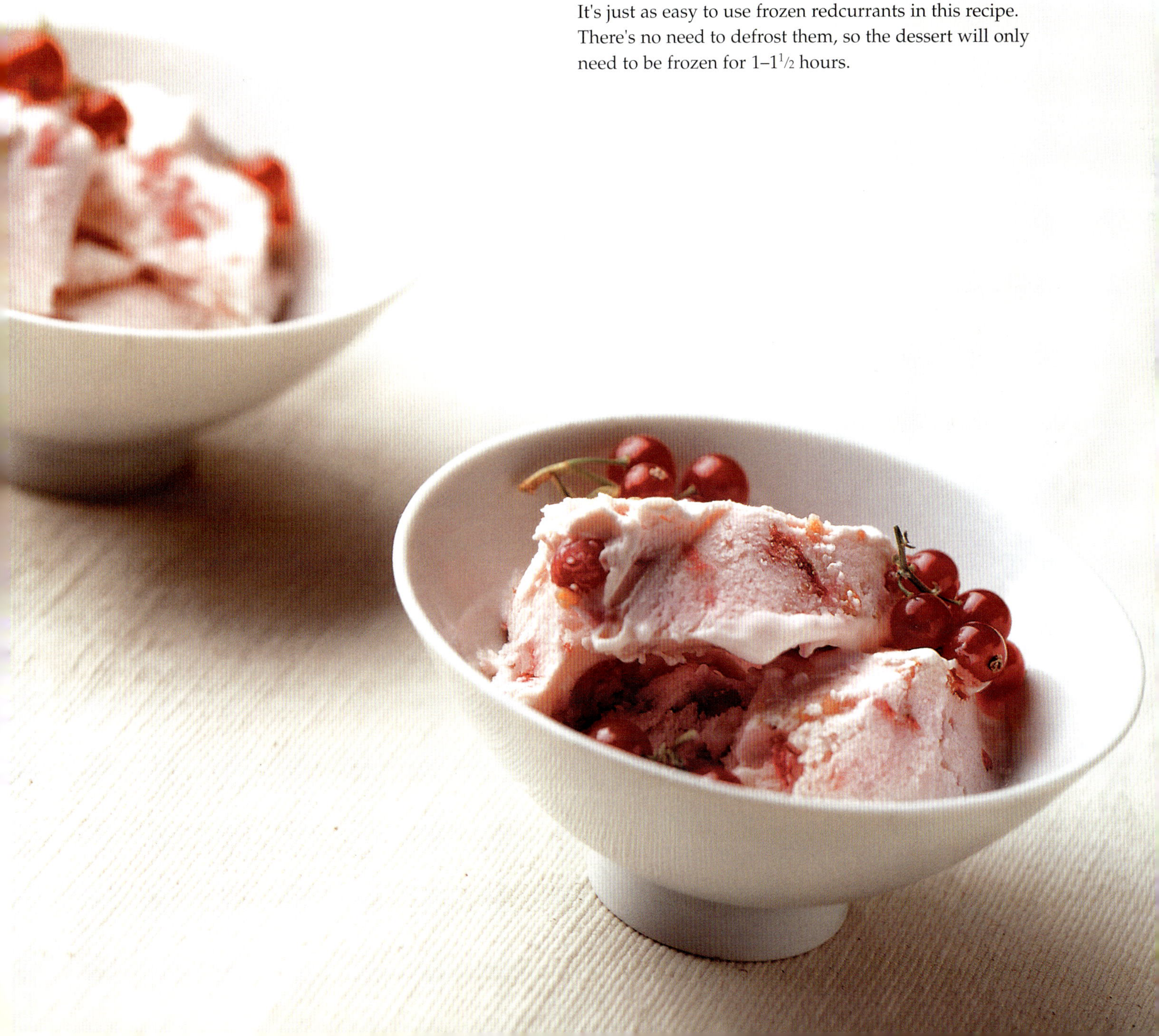

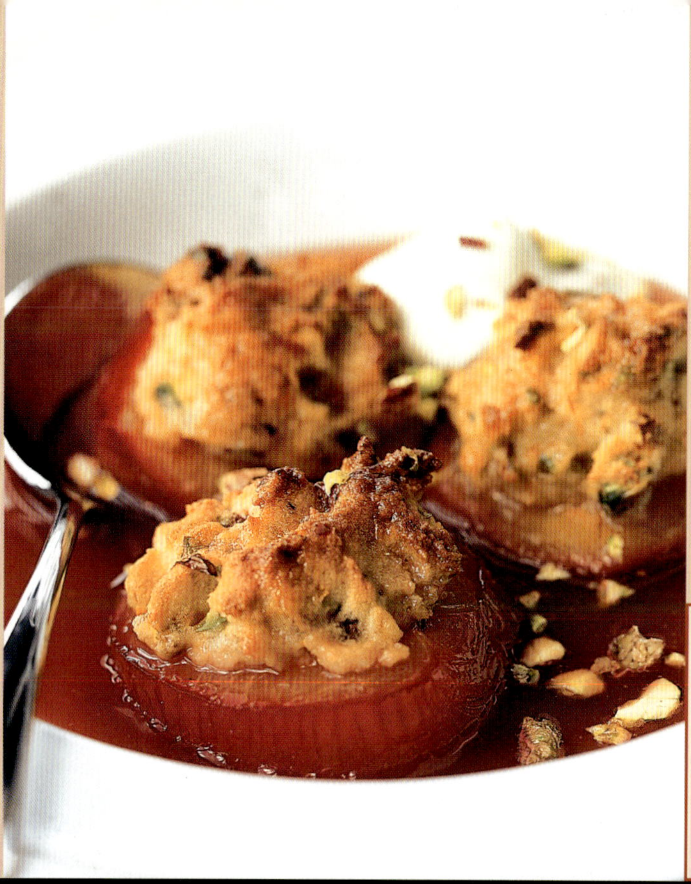

**PER SERVING**
215 kcalories
protein 7g
carbohydrate 23g
fat 11g
saturated fat 1g
fibre 3g
added sugar 8g
salt 0.11g

## Facts about fibre

*When it was called 'roughage', it seemed like it was always a good thing, now it's referred to as 'fibre', it's all a bit more complex, with potential drawbacks, and it doesn't seem like the same simple story. What are the facts about fibre?*

**What exactly is fibre and what does it do?**

*Some of the more complex forms of carbohydrates, like those that form the plant cell walls, etc. (mainly cellulose), simply cannot be digested and so pass through our digestive system virtually unchanged – we call it dietary fibre or roughage – but, in so doing, it performs the important function of helping the speedy and efficient passage of all material through the system. As well as staving off intestinal problems like diverticulitis and bowel cancer, it also helps us feel full. Some soluble forms of fibre are even credited with helping lower blood LDL ('bad') cholesterol (see page 94) and they help stabilize blood sugar levels.*

**Can too much fibre ever be harmful?**

*Some foods that are particularly rich in insoluble fibre, like wheat bran, can interfere with the process of absorbing nutrients from other foods present in the digestive system at the same time (say the calcium in the milk with a cereal). It is, therefore, much healthier to find your fibre from whole foods that are naturally high in fibre, like beans or wholemeal bread, than in manufactured products like bran supplements and bran-enriched breakfast cereals.*

**How do I ensure I am getting enough fibre?**

*If you are eating plenty of fruit and veg – your 'five a day' then you are probably well on your way there! Beans and other pulses are among the richest sources, as are wholemeal bread and pasta – and oats, of course, in the form of either porridge or muesli. Dried fruit, nuts and seeds make the best snacks if your are trying to boost your fibre intake.*

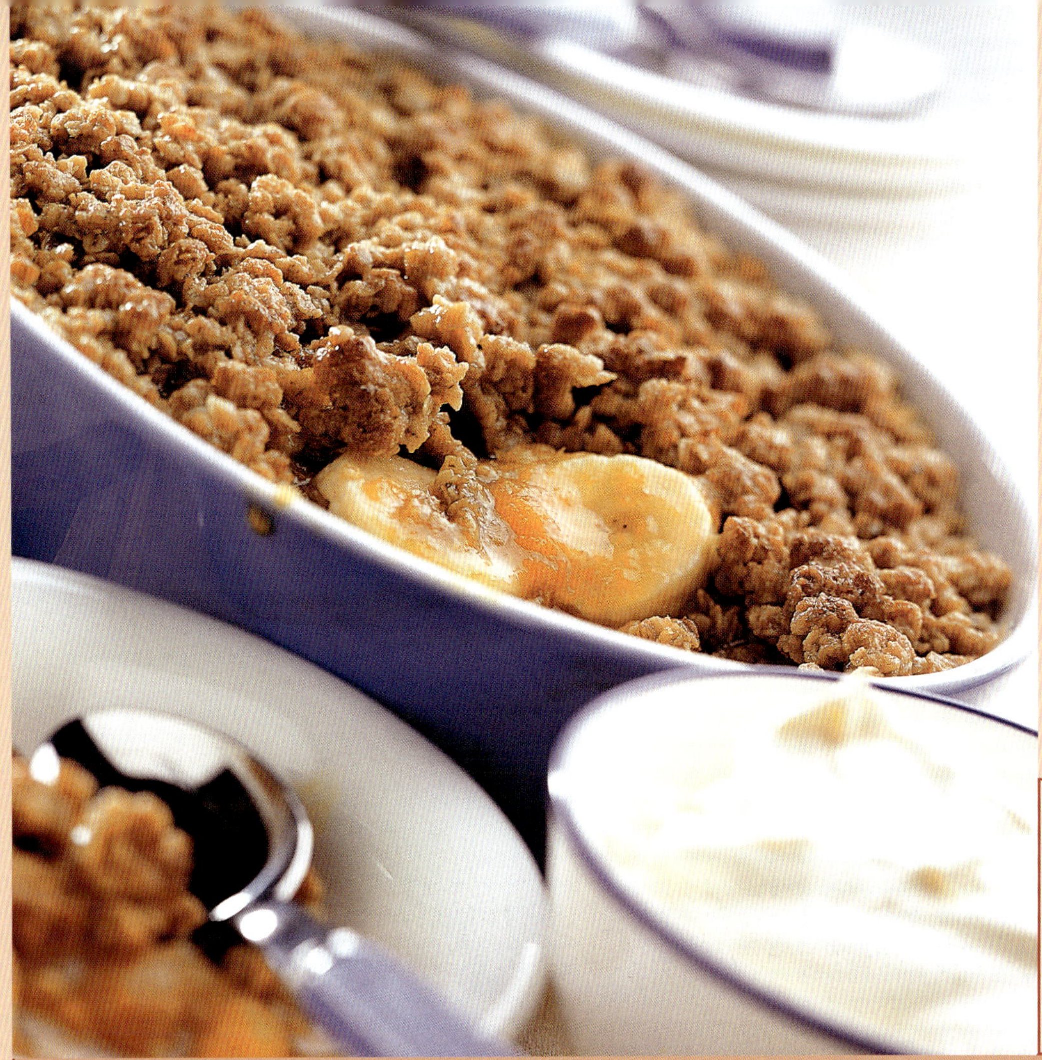

PER SERVING
189 kcalories
protein 6g
carbohydrate 19g
fat 10g
saturated fat 1g
fibre 2g
added sugar 8g
salt 0.09g

**Lots of lovely sweet treats can be abundant sources of fibre ▼**

## Apricot Flapjack Crumble

*(above) needs an oven preheated to 190°C/375°F/Gas 5. Spread out 600g/1¼ lb jar of apricot compote and 4 unpeeled and sliced bananas, each about 150g/5oz, in a 1.5-litre/2¾-pint shallow ovenproof dish.*

*Heat 70g/2½oz butter, 85g/3oz light muscovado sugar and 1 tablespoon golden syrup in a pan over a low heat. When the butter has melted, stir in 150g/5oz porridge oats and 2 tablespoons plain flour. Spoon the mixture over the fruit, and spread gently with a fork.*

*Bake for 20 minutes until the top is golden and firm. Allow to cool slightly, then serve with cream or custard.*

## Pistachio Plums with Orange Syrup

*(opposite) again requires an oven preheated to 190°C/375°F/Gas 5. Lay 6 large halved and stoned plums, cut side up, in a shallow oven-proof dish. Put the whites of 2 eggs in a bowl and whisk until foamy. Using a metal spoon, stir 30g/1oz unsalted shelled pistachios, roughly chopped (reserving 1 tablespoon), into the egg white, together with 50g/2oz ground almonds, 1 tablespoon caster sugar and the grated zest of 1 large orange.*

*Pile the nut mixture into the plum halves. Pour the juice of 2 large oranges around them and sprinkle with a tablespoon of Amaretto, if you like, and 1 tablespoon muscovado sugar. Bake for 30 minutes, basting occasionally with the orange juice.*

*Serve the plums hot, with the orange syrup spooned around them. Sprinkle with the reserved pistachios and add a spoonful of fat-free fromage frais.*

# Fried Rum Bananas

**Bananas really are a very healthy food; rich in vitamins and minerals, especially B6 and potassium, they are also a great source of fibre - and a good source of slowly released energy.**

PREPARATION 2 minutes
COOKING 6–7 minutes

a knob of butter
4 bananas, sliced at an angle into 4 pieces
4 tbsp rum or brandy
4 tbsp double cream or crème fraîche
2 tbsp light muscovado sugar

1 Melt the butter in a large frying pan. When it is foaming, fry the bananas for 2 minutes, then turn them and pour in the rum or brandy. Fry for 1–2 minutes more until browned.
2 Stir the cream or crème fraîche and sugar into the pan and warm through for 1 minute.
3 Divide the bananas between 4 plates and spoon over the sauce. Serve immediately.

PER SERVING
**237 kcalories**
**protein 2g**
**carbohydrate 32g**
**fat 9g**
**saturated fat 5g**
**fibre 1g**
**added sugar 8g**
**salt 0.11g**

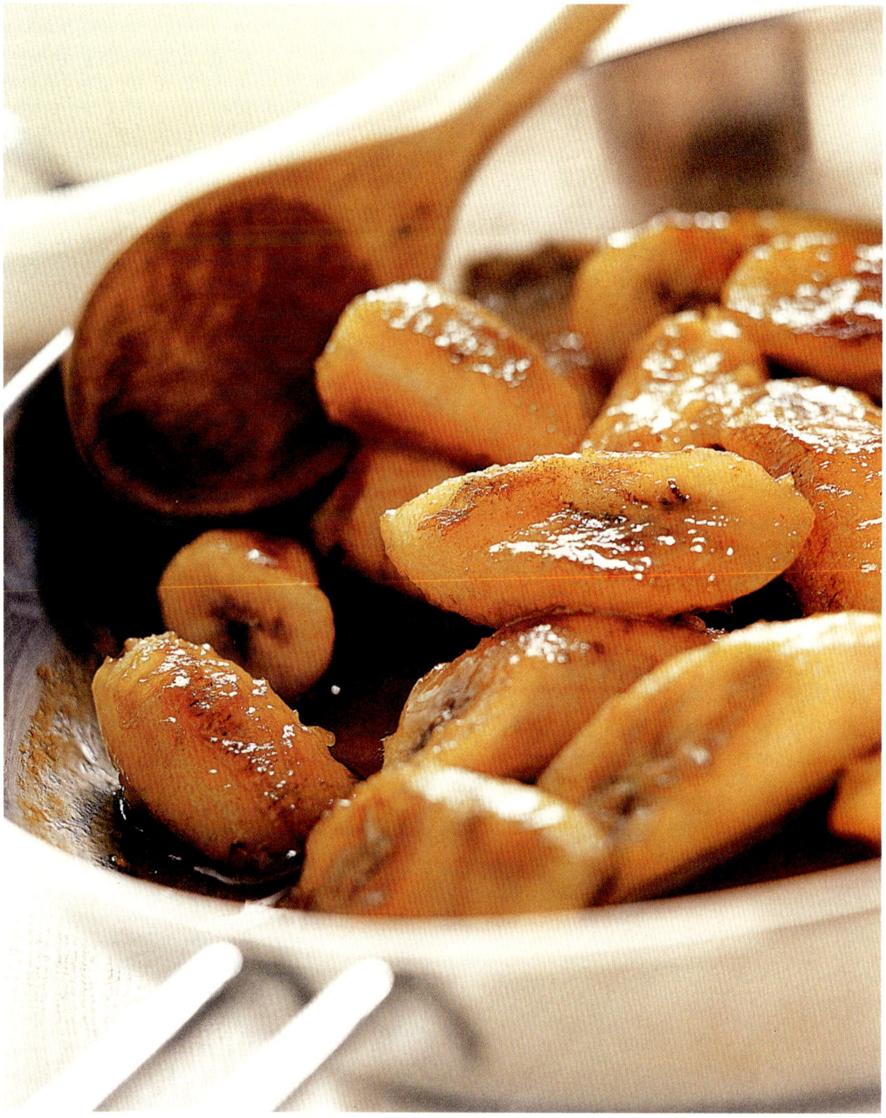

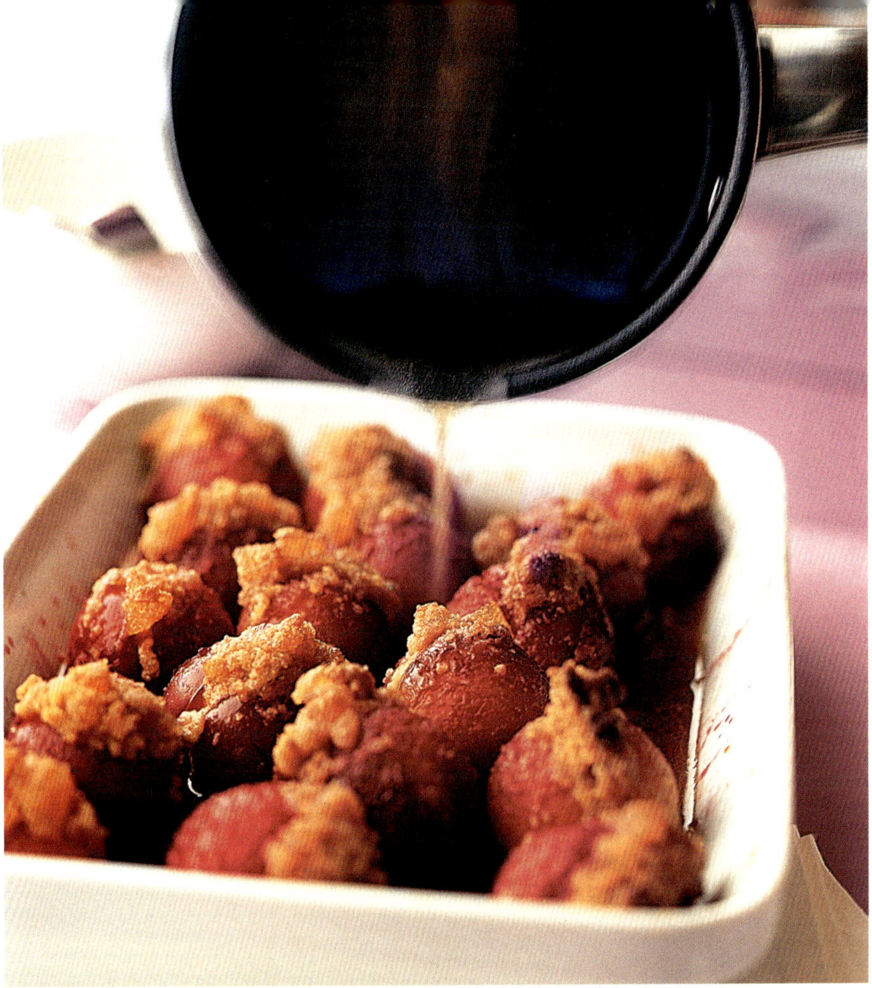

PER SERVING
263 kcalories
protein 1g
carbohydrate 43g
fat 8g
saturated fat 5g
fibre 2g
added sugar 28g
salt 0.33g

# Roast Brandy Plums with Ginger

**Any kind of plum can be roasted in this way. Apricots and peaches are equally delicious.**

SERVES 6
PREPARATION 20 minutes
COOKING 10–15 minutes

750g/1lb 10oz plums
125ml/4fl oz blackcurrant cordial, such as Ribena
4 tbsp brandy
ice-cream or thick cream, to serve

**for the stuffing**

50g/2oz dry biscuits, such as Rich Tea
50g/2oz butter, at room temperature
50g/2oz demerara sugar
50g/2oz candied or crystallized ginger, chopped

1 Preheat the oven to 200°C/400°F/Gas 6. Rinse the plums and pat them dry. Run a knife halfway along their indentation, then scoop out the stones and discard.

2 Make the stuffing: crumble the biscuits with your fingers, or crush them in a bowl with the end of a rolling pin. Using an electric mixer, cream the butter with the sugar, then stir in the biscuit crumbs and the chopped ginger.

3 Push small mounds of the stuffing into the plums. Set them in a baking dish and spoon over the blackcurrant cordial. Roast the plums in the oven, basting regularly, until they are tender and one or two skins have split; this should take about 10–15 minutes depending on their size and ripeness. (When they're out of season and fairly unripe, the plums can take up to 30 minutes to cook.)

4 Remove the plums from the oven. Heat the brandy in a small pan until it just starts to bubble. Set it alight – use a long taper and stand back from the flames. Pour the flaming brandy over the plums.

5 Serve hot with ice-cream or at room temperature with thick cream.

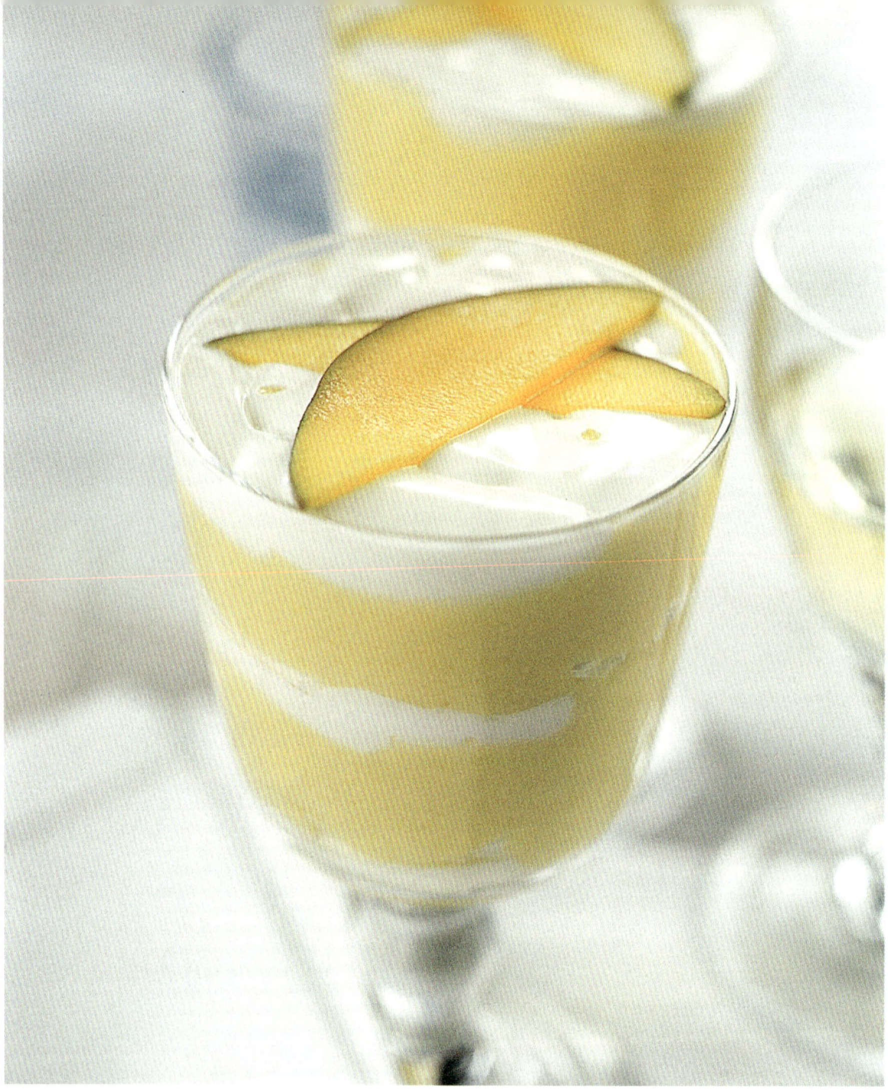

# Mango Meringue Fool

PER SERVING
302 kcalories
protein 8g
carbohydrate 47g
fat 10g
saturated fat 6g
fibre 3g
added sugar 30g
salt 0.56g

**Mangoes are 'superfoods' (see page 100), being the richest fruit source of the protective carotenoids and with lots of antioxidant vitamin E.**

PREPARATION 15 minutes

1 large ripe mango
125g/4½oz carton of low-fat soft cheese
30g/1oz icing sugar
4 meringue nests
200ml/7fl oz carton of half-fat crème fraîche

1 Peel the skin from the mango thinly with a sharp knife, then slice the thick wedge of flesh off each side, cutting right to the stone. Cut off the rest of the flesh as best you can (it's impossible to be tidy). Cut 8 thin slices and reserve, then whiz the rest in a food processor until smooth. In a bowl, beat the cheese and sugar, then gradually beat in the mango purée.
2 Crumble the meringue, then layer up with the mango fool and crème fraîche in glass tumblers.
3 Decorate with mango slices and chill until ready to serve.

# Fragrant Rosé Peaches

PER SERVING
239 kcalories
protein 2g
carbohydrate 40g
fat 8g
saturated fat 5g
fibre 2g
added sugar 30g
salt 0.03g

**White-fleshed peaches are the sweetest and juiciest, and tend to be more expensive than the yellow-fleshed variety. They are not so easily available but are worth spending a little extra on when you can find them. You can substitute nectarines in any recipe that uses skinned peaches.**

PREPARATION 10 minutes, plus about 1 hour cooling
COOKING 10 minutes

75cl bottle of light fruity rosé wine (such as Cabernet d'Anjou)
100g/4oz caster sugar
4 peaches
4 tbsp crème fraîche
handful of small fresh mint leaves, to decorate

1 Put the wine and sugar in a large pan and stir over a gentle heat until the sugar has dissolved. Increase the heat and boil rapidly for 10 minutes until the liquid has reduced by about one-third. Transfer to a bowl to cool, then cover and chill until completely cold (this will take about 30 minutes).
2 Meanwhile, skin the peaches, then cut them in half and remove the stones. Cut into slices about 5mm/¼in thick and divide between 4 serving bowls.
3 Add a tablespoon of crème fraîche to each serving, then pour in the rosé syrup. Scatter over the mint leaves and serve immediately.

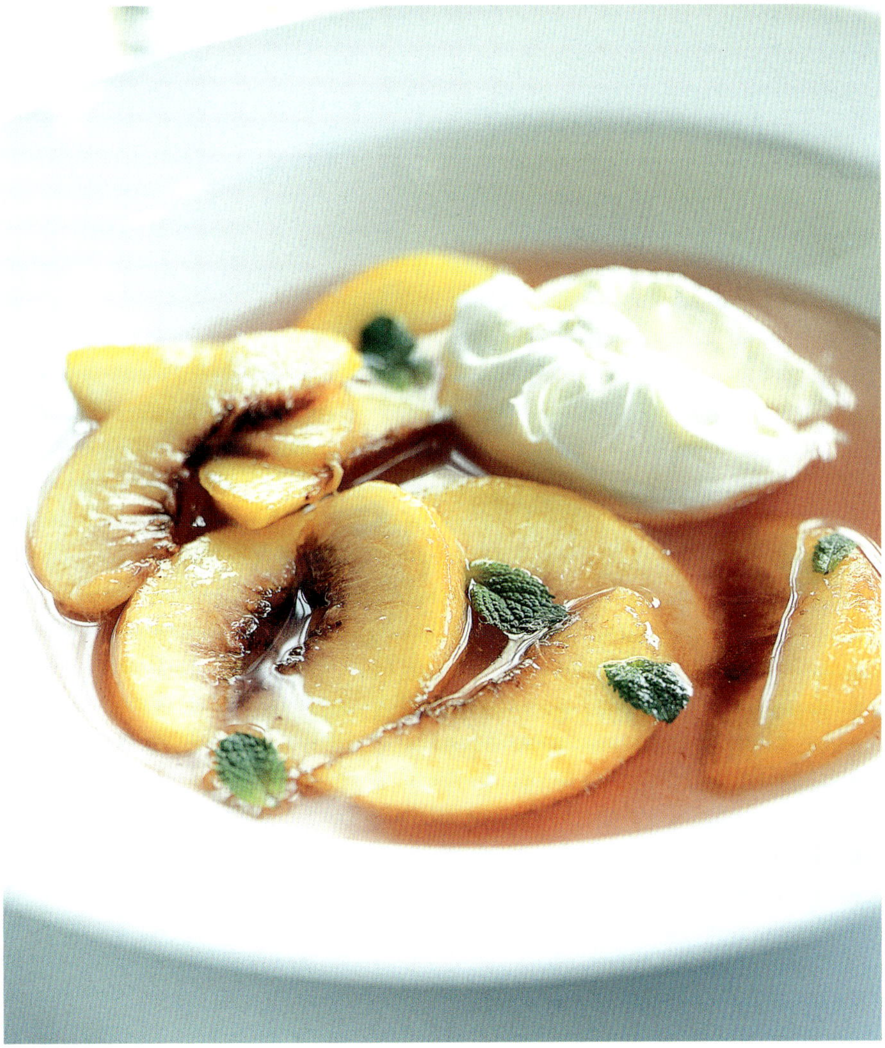

# Lemon Sponge Drops

**PER SERVING**
**225 kcalories**
**protein 9g**
**carbohydrate 38g**
**fat 4g**
**saturated fat 1g**
**fibre trace**
**added sugar 22g**
**salt 0.15g**

**Fat-free sponges are great for desserts, and this one is really quick to put together. The sponge drops in this recipe are softened with a lemon syrup, making them plump and moist.**

PREPARATION 10 minutes
COOKING 15 minutes

- 2 large eggs, separated
- 85g/3oz golden caster sugar
- grated zest and juice of 1 lemon
- 50g/2oz plain flour
- 2 tbsp orange-flavoured liqueur, such as Cointreau or Grand Marnier
- 200g/7oz carton of fat-free fromage frais, to serve
- ground cinnamon, to dust

1 Preheat the oven to 180°C/350°F/Gas 4. In a bowl, whisk together the egg whites and 30g/1oz of the sugar until the mixture forms soft peaks. Add another 30g/1oz sugar, the lemon zest and egg yolks, and whisk until well blended. Gently fold in the flour.

2 Spoon the mixture into a greased four-hole Yorkshire pudding tin (each recess about 9cm/3½in wide) or a flexible rubber muffin mould. Bake for 10 minutes until risen, golden and firm to the touch.

3 Meanwhile, put the remaining sugar in a small pan with 200ml/7fl oz water and the lemon juice. Slowly bring to the boil, stirring until the sugar has dissolved. Pour into a heatproof bowl and stir in the liqueur.

4 When the sponge drops are cooked, remove from the tin and sit them in a shallow dish. Pour over the warm syrup and allow them to cool to room temperature. This gives the lemon syrup time to soak into the sponges.

5 Divide the sponges between serving plates and top with a spoonful of fromage frais. Dust with a little ground cinnamon and serve.

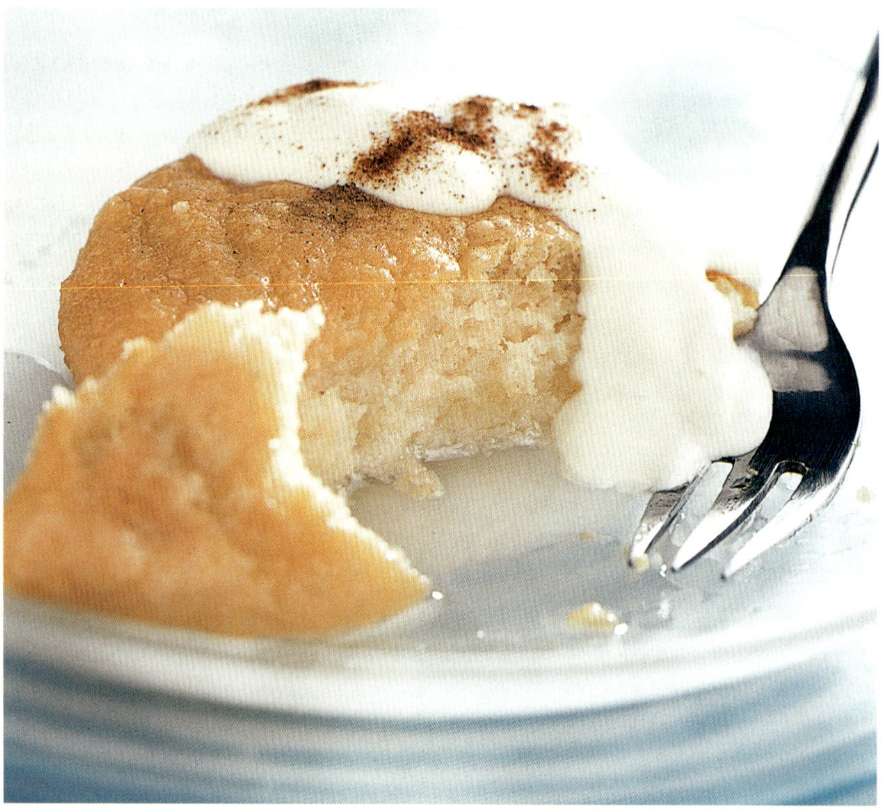

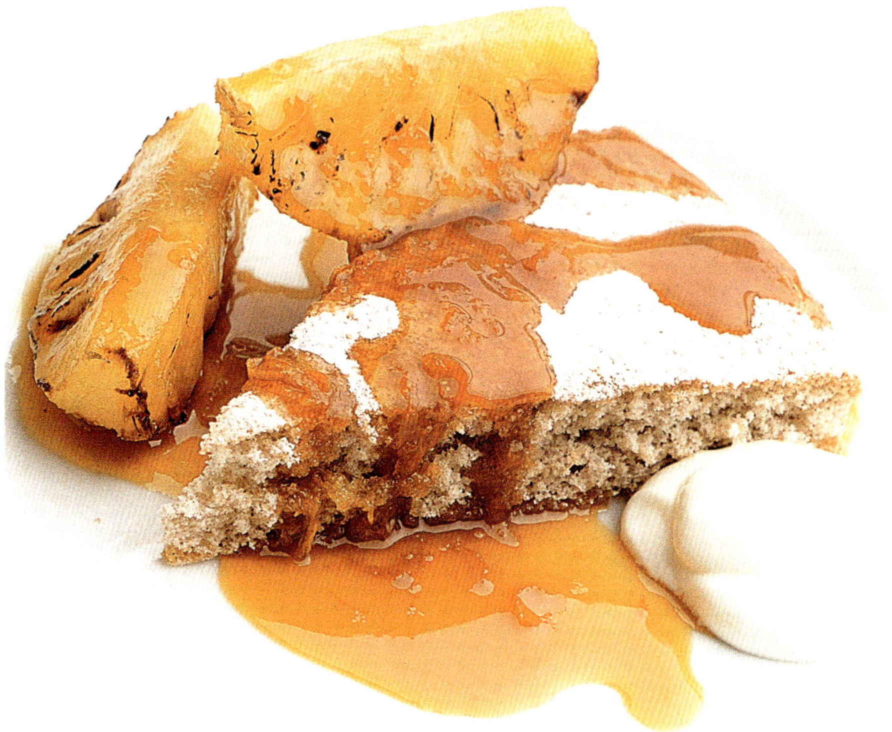

# Cinnamon Cake and Caramelized Pineapple with Rum Sauce

PER SERVING
193 kcalories
protein 4g
carbohydrate 35g
fat 3g
saturated fat 1g
fibre 1g
added sugar 17g
salt 0.08g

**As the cake is made without any fat, it doesn't keep well - eat it all on the day it is made or freeze leftovers. If you can't find baby pineapples, cut a larger one into 12 longer, thinner wedges. Cinnamon is a powerful natural decongestant.**

SERVES 6
PREPARATION 30 minutes
COOKING 30–35 minutes

vegetable oil, for greasing
a little plain flour, for dusting
2 eggs
50g/2oz caster sugar
50g/2oz plain flour
1 tsp ground cinnamon
icing sugar, for dusting

**for the sauce**
grated zest of 1 orange
juice of 4 oranges (equivalent to 300ml/$^1/_2$ pint fresh orange juice)
4 tbsp dark rum
2 tbsp clear honey

**for the caramelized pineapple**
2 baby pineapples, peeled and each cut into 6 wedges
2 tsp caster sugar

1 Preheat the oven to 180°C/350°F/Gas 4 and lightly grease a round 20cm/8in cake tin. Tip in a little flour and rotate the tin to coat base and sides. Shake out any excess.
2 In a large mixing bowl, whisk the eggs and sugar until the mixture forms a trail on the surface when you lift out the beaters (about 5 minutes). Sift over the flour and cinnamon and carefully fold these in using a large metal spoon.
3 Pour the mixture into the tin and bake for 15–20 minutes, until pale golden and spongy to the touch. Let it cool for a few minutes, then turn out on to a wire rack.
4 Make the sauce: in a pan, bring all the ingredients to the boil, then boil rapidly for 5 minutes until the sauce is reduced by about one-third. Allow to cool to a thin syrup-like consistency before serving.
5 Preheat the grill to hot. Pat the pineapple wedges dry and lay on a baking sheet. Sprinkle with the caster sugar and grill for 3–4 minutes, until they begin to turn golden brown. Turn and grill for another 2–3 minutes.
6 Cut the cake into 6 wedges and lightly dust each piece with icing sugar before setting on serving plates. Put 2 caramelized pineapple wedges to the side of each cake slice, then drizzle over the rum sauce and serve.

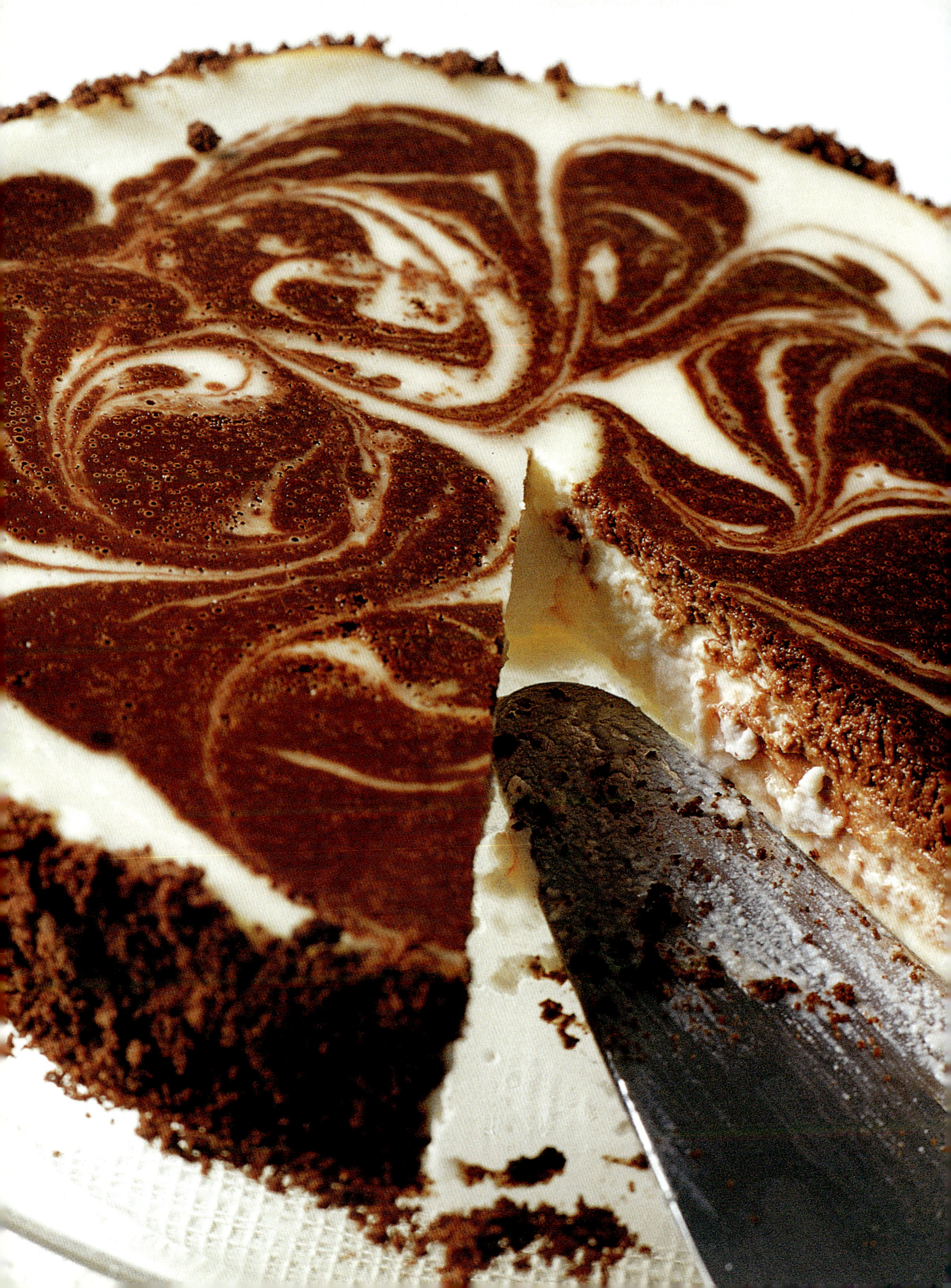

# Chocolate Marble Cheesecake

**Chocolate really isn't the evil it's made out to be; it is generally the things that are added to it - lots of sugar, eggs and dairy fat - that cause the problems. In fact, chocolate itself is a valuable source of antioxidants and iron. Here and in the recipes on pages 131 and 134 judicious use of low-fat cheeses, yoghurt, skimmed milk, egg whites in place of whole eggs and not too much added sugar produce splendid chocolate feasts that are full of flavour but not cloying. You can make your own chocolate cookies for a dark crunchy case, or substitute bought low-fat ones.**

PER SERVING
**229 kcalories**
**protein 12g**
**carbohydrate 29g**
**fat 8g**
**saturated fat 2g**
**fibre 1g**
**added sugar 24g**
**salt 1.04g**

SERVES 10
PREPARATION 20–25 minutes, plus cooling and chilling (at least 12 hours)
COOKING 40 minutes

clean-tasting vegetable oil, for greasing
two 250g/9oz cartons of low-fat (less than 2%) cottage cheese
200g/7oz carton of light soft cheese, at room temperature
3 eggs
200g/7oz caster sugar, plus 1 tbsp
1 tbsp vanilla extract
1½ tsp lemon juice
½ tsp salt
3 tbsp cocoa powder
2 tsp instant espresso or coffee powder
4 Chocolate Cookies (see page 131)

1 Preheat the oven to 180°C/350°F/Gas 4 and lightly oil the sides of a 20cm/8in round cake tin (not loose-based) that is 4cm/1½in deep. Line the base with greaseproof paper.
2 Blend the cottage cheese in a food processor for 2–3 minutes until smooth, scraping it down the sides of the bowl when necessary. Add the soft cheese with the eggs, 200g/7oz caster sugar, the vanilla, lemon juice and salt. Pulse until perfectly smooth. Do not overprocess.
3 Whisk the cocoa powder, coffee powder, remaining 1 tablespoon of caster sugar and 3 tablespoons cold water in a large bowl until smooth, then stir in 200ml/7fl oz of the cheesecake mixture until smooth.
4 Spoon three-quarters of the remaining cheesecake mixture into the cake tin. Spoon the chocolate batter into the centre, then spoon the remaining plain batter into the centre of the chocolate batter. Using a table knife, make circular strokes to marble the batters until nicely but not completely mingled.
5 Stand the cake tin in a roasting tin about 5cm/2in deep and 5cm/2in wider than the cake tin. Slide the lower shelf out of the oven slightly and put the roasting tin on it. Pour boiling water into the roasting tin to a depth of 2.5cm/1in, then carefully slide the shelf back.
6 Bake the cheesecake until slightly risen and just beginning to shrink from the edges of the cake tin, about 40 minutes. Transfer the cake tin to a wire rack and leave to cool. Cover with cling film and chill for at least 12 hours or up to one day before serving.
7 To serve, put a flat plate on top of the cling film. Invert the two and tap the tin until the cheesecake is released. Peel away the greaseproof paper, then invert the cheesecake on to a serving plate and peel away the cling film. Finely crush the cookies in a plastic bag with a rolling pin, then press them around the sides of the cheesecake using a palette knife and your fingers. Slice using a sharp thin knife, dipping the knife in hot water and wiping dry after each slice.

# Pancakes with Hot Passion Fruit Sauce

**PER SERVING**
**140 kcalories**
**protein 5g**
**carbohydrate 23g**
**fat 4g**
**saturated fat 1g**
**fibre 2g**
**added sugar 3g**
**salt 0.13g**

**This is a lighter, more fragrant version of crêpes Suzette.**

PREPARATION 25 minutes
COOKING about 25 minutes

- 50g/2oz plain flour
- 1 egg
- 150ml/¼ pint semi-skimmed milk
- grated zest of 1 orange
- 2 tsp groundnut oil, for frying
- 300ml/½ pint good-quality orange juice
- 1 tbsp muscovado sugar
- 4 passion fruit, halved with the pulp scooped out
- 100g/4oz fresh raspberries

1 Tip the flour into a large bowl. Make a well in the centre and crack in the egg. Gradually whisk in the milk to form a smooth batter, then stir in the orange zest.
2 Heat a small non-stick frying pan. Add a little oil, then wipe out the pan with kitchen paper. Pour enough batter into the pan just to coat the base, then cook for about 1 minute. Loosen the edges with a spatula, then turn (or toss) the pancake and cook the other side. Continue until you have 8 thin pancakes; set aside.
3 Pour the orange juice and sugar into the pan. Bring to the boil and simmer for 5 minutes until slightly reduced. Stir in the passion fruit pulp.
4 Gently fold each pancake in half, then in half again to make triangles; slide into the hot orange and passion fruit sauce to warm through.
5 Serve at once with the fresh raspberries.

# 30-minute Summer Pudding

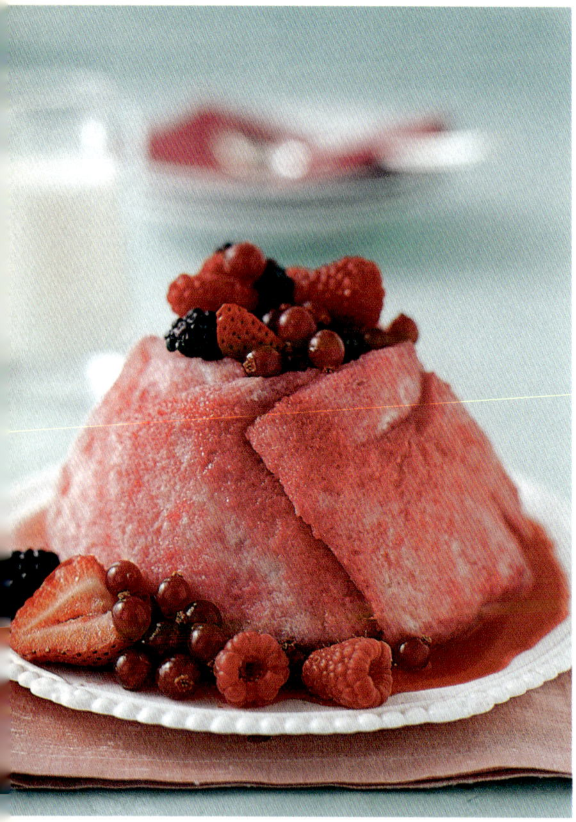

SERVES 6
PREPARATION about 30 minutes
COOKING about 15 minutes

- 100g/4oz caster sugar
- 900g/2lb mixture of summer fruits, such as hulled strawberries, raspberries, red and blackcurrants, blackberries, cherries
- 8-9 thin slices white bread from a small unsliced sandwich tin loaf, crusts removed
- cream, to serve

**PER SERVING**
**221 kcalories • protein 5g • carbohydrate 51g fat 1g • saturated fat none • fibre 4g added sugar 18g • salt 0.63g**

1 Put sugar and 125ml/4fl oz water in a large pan with all the fruits except the strawberries and raspberries. Stir over moderate heat to dissolve sugar. Remove from heat. Cut any large strawberries in half, then add to the sugar syrup with the raspberries. Gently stir; set aside for 10 minutes.
2 Drain fruits from juice. Using 6–7 slices of bread, dip each briefly in juice to coat and line a 1.2 litre/2 pint basin overlapping slices around the sides (leave bottom uncovered).
3 Reserve a spoonful of cooked fruits, then, using a slotted spoon, spoon rest into basin, pressing down as you go so they are well packed and filling right to the top. Spoon a little juice over. Press remaining slices of bread over top of fruits, trimming to fit. Spoon over a little more juice.
4 Loosen sides with a knife and invert on a plate. Spoon reserved cooked fruits into top and pour over the remaining juices. Scatter a few fresh fruits around and serve with cream.

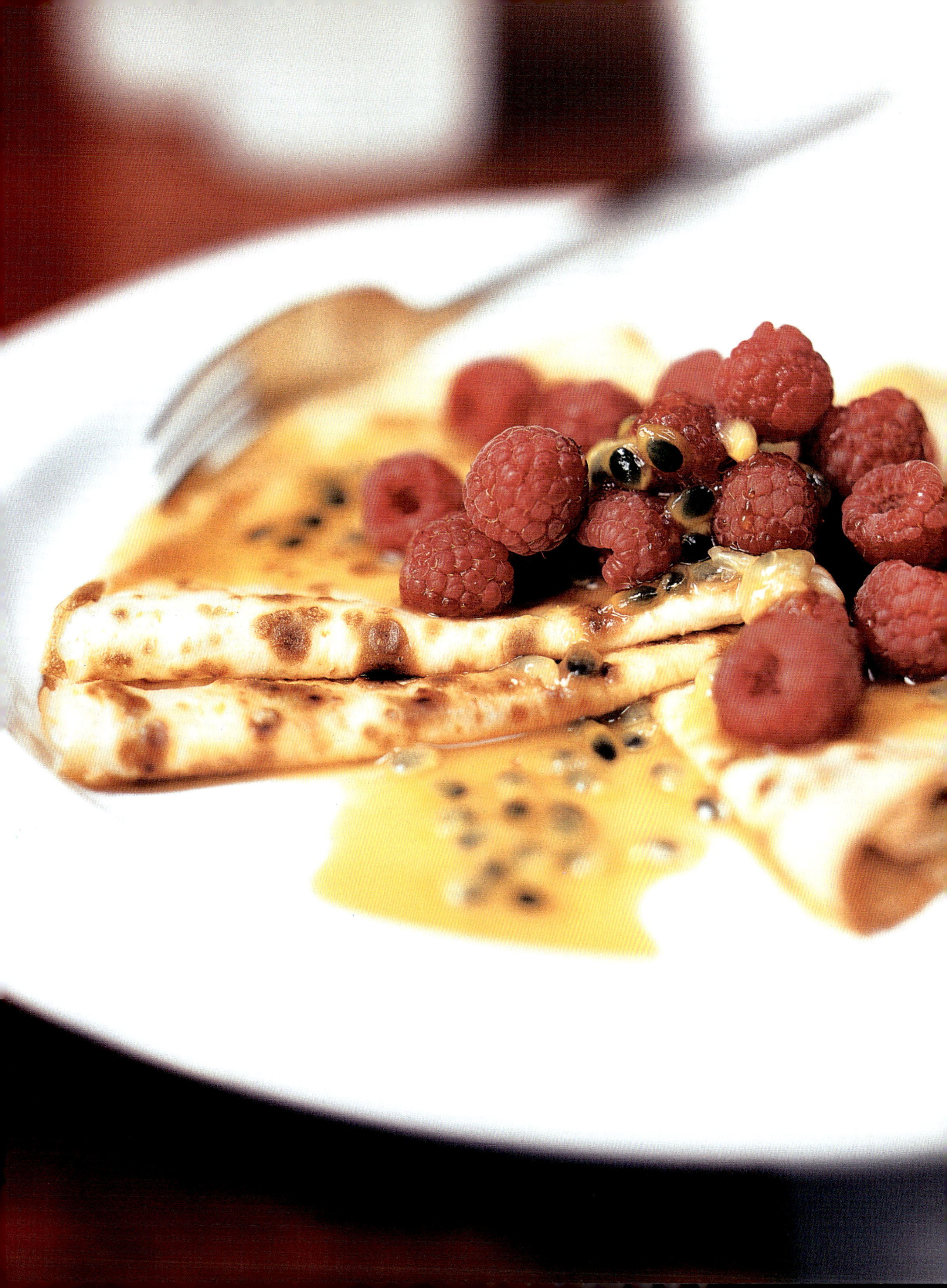

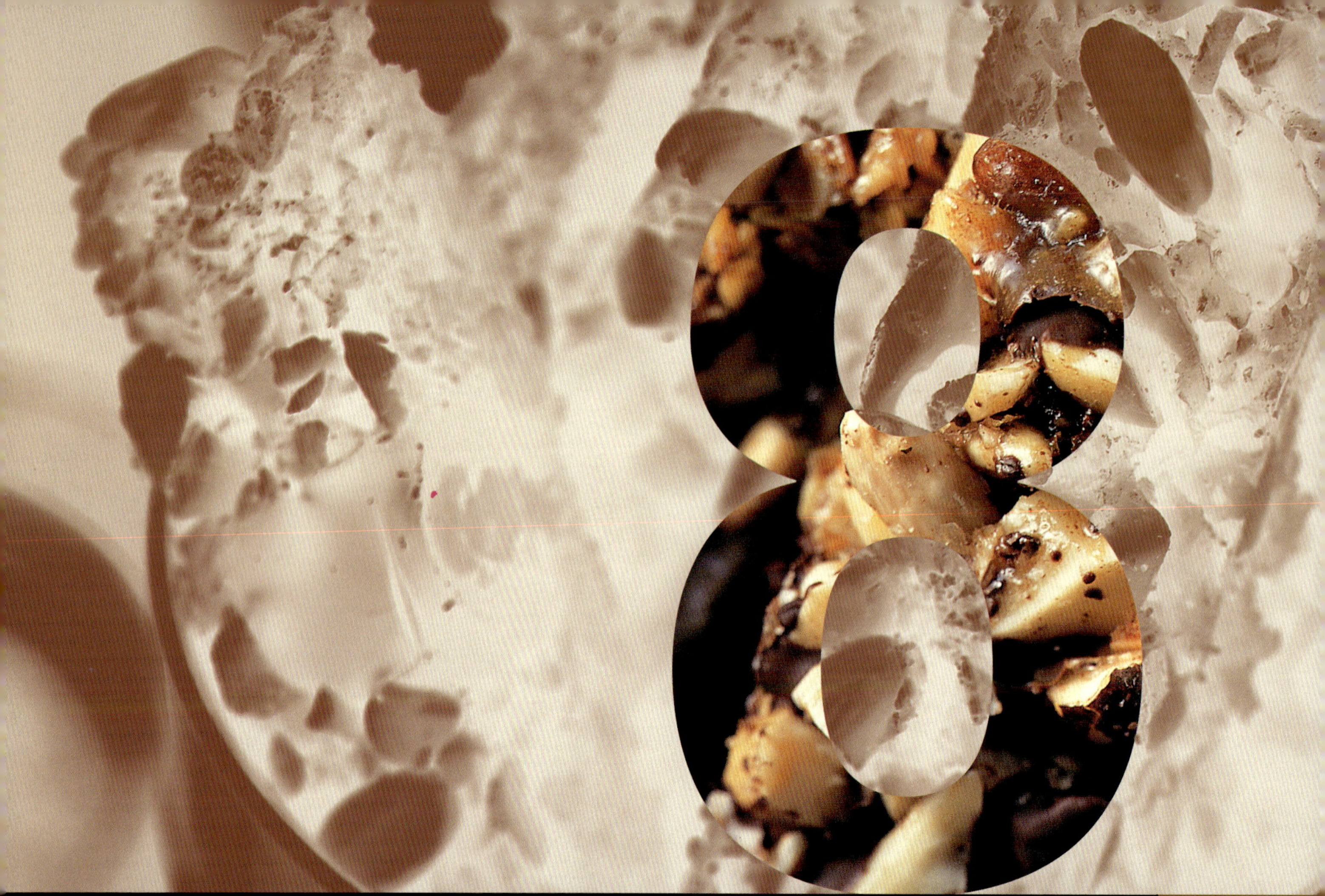


# Balanced Bakes

*Because of high added-sugar levels, baking is again one of those areas that those concerned with healthy eating tend to avoid. It is, however, an excellent way of getting into the diet more of some important 'superfoods' (see page 100) like apples, oranges, carrots, oats, nuts and seeds, as well as other healthy – if not quite in the 'super' league – goodies like dried fruit and bananas. More importantly, everyone craves a sweet indulgence from time to time, and it is much better that you enjoy something like the merit-packed delights on the following pages than buying really oversweetened, positively unhealthy and relatively expensive commercial sweets, nuts and chocolate bars.*

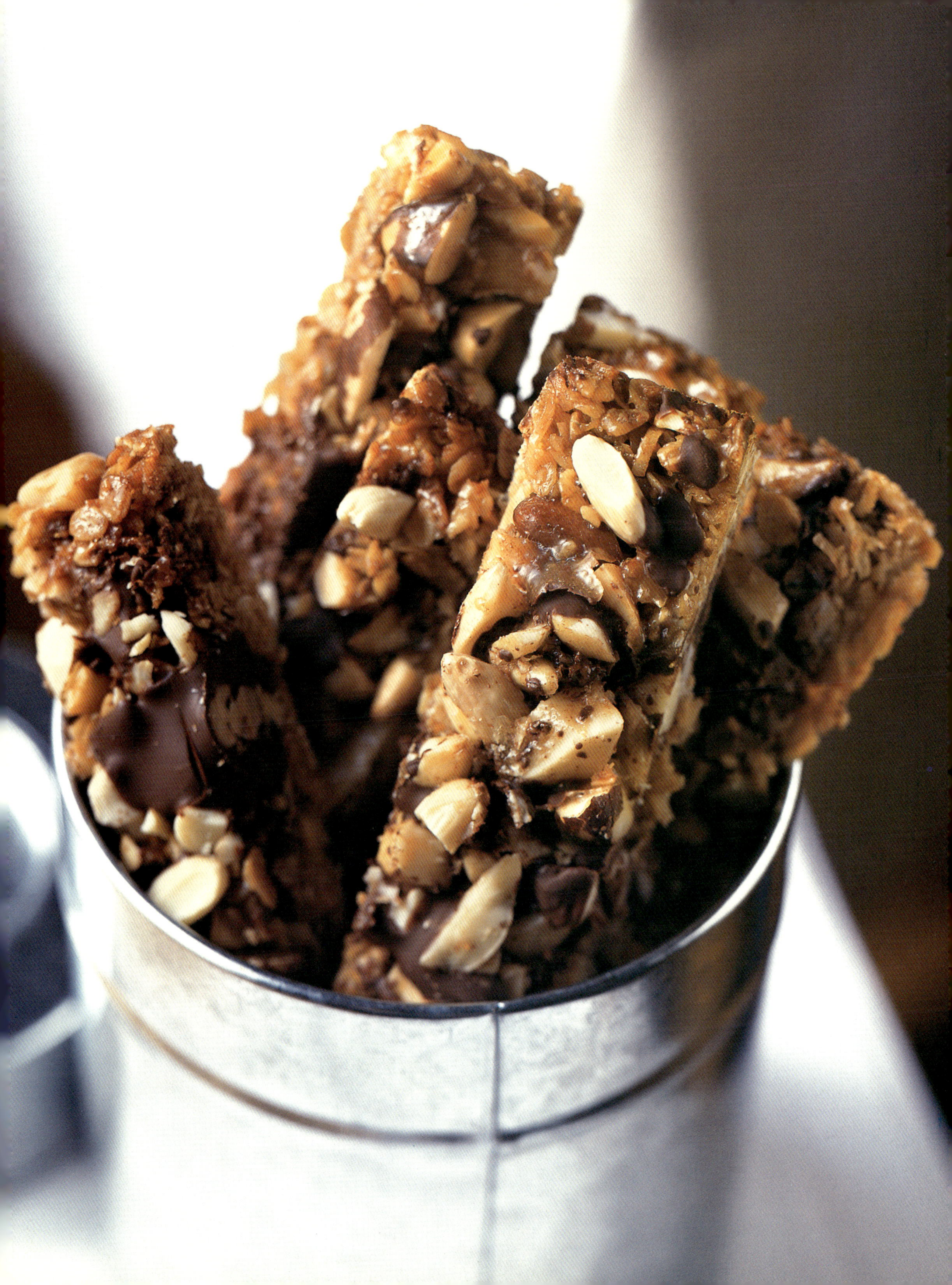

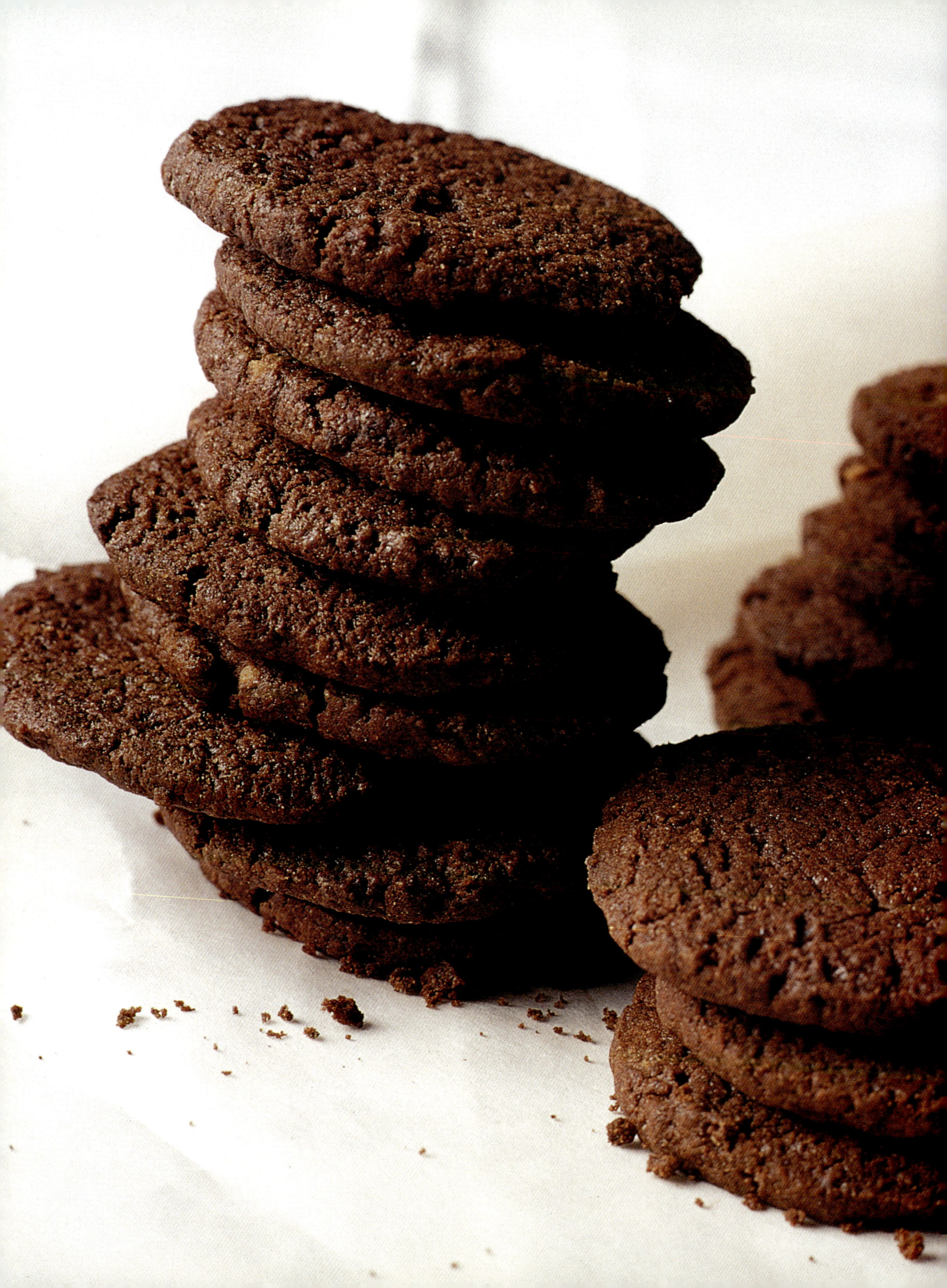

# Chunky Chocolate Nut Flapjacks

PER FLAPJACK
325 kcalories
protein 5g
carbohydrate 28g
fat 22g
saturated fat 10g
fibre 2g
added sugar 15g
salt 0.3g

**These flapjacks bulge with chunks of chocolate and nuts, so a little goes a long way. It's good in any healthy regime to allow yourself the occasional treat. However, Brazil nuts, cashews, almonds and oats are all 'superfoods' (see page 100); so, with their moderate added fat and sugar content, these scrummy bars are almost too good for you to be true.**

MAKES 12
PREPARATION 15 minutes
COOKING about 30 minutes

200g/7oz oats
30g/1oz desiccated coconut
150g/5oz butter, cut into pieces
50g/2oz light muscovado sugar
5 tbsp golden syrup
100g/4oz Brazil nuts or cashews, cut into large chunks
50g/2oz almonds, cut into large chunks
85g/3oz good-quality dark chocolate, cut into large chunks

1 Preheat the oven to 180°C/350°F/Gas 4. Lightly butter a 23cm/9in square shallow baking tin about 4cm/1½in deep. Line the base with baking parchment if the tin is not non-stick. Mix together the oats and coconut.
2 Put the butter, sugar and syrup in a pan. Cook over a low heat, stirring occasionally, until the butter has melted and the sugar dissolved. Remove from the heat and stir in the oat-and-coconut mixture. Spoon into the tin and press down evenly. Scatter over the nuts and press lightly into the mixture. Stick the chunks of chocolate between the nuts. Bake for 25–30 minutes, or until pale golden.
3 Mark the bars or squares with the back of a knife while the mixture is still warm, then allow to cool completely before cutting through and removing from the tin.

# Chocolate Cookies

PER COOKIE
78 kcalories
protein 1g
carbohydrate 10g
fat 4g
saturated fat 2g
fibre none
added sugar 6g
salt 0.18g

**Cookies baked for a little less time will be crisp outside and slightly soft within. Bake a little longer for dry, crisp, tender ones. The softer ones dry out after a day or so.**

MAKES 25
PREPARATION 20–25 minutes, plus chilling
COOKING 14 minutes

140g/5oz plain flour
50g/2oz cocoa powder
¼ tsp bicarbonate of soda
¼ tsp salt
50g/2oz plus 1 tbsp light soft brown sugar
50g/2oz plus 1 tbsp white granulated sugar
50g/2oz unsalted butter, at room temperature
50g/2oz margarine
1 tsp vanilla extract
white of 1 egg

1 Combine the flour, cocoa powder, bicarbonate of soda and salt, and mix well. Combine the sugars, mixing well with the fingers to press out any lumps. If the lumps are stubborn, put in the food processor for a few seconds.
2 Beat the butter and margarine with an electric whisk or wooden spoon until creamy. Tip in the flour and sugar mixtures, the vanilla and egg white. Beat to form a dough, then shape into a 25cm/10in long log. Wrap in cling film and chill for 45 minutes or until needed.
3 Preheat the oven to 180°C/350°F/Gas 4 and line 2 heavy baking sheets with non-stick baking parchment or foil. Slice off rounds of dough, each about 5mm/¼in thick, and place about 2.5cm/1in apart on the baking sheets. Bake for 14 minutes. (If necessary, swap the sheets halfway or bake the ones on the lower shelves for a little longer.) The cookies will puff and crackle on top, and settle when done.
4 Using a spatula, transfer the cookies to a wire rack and leave to cool.

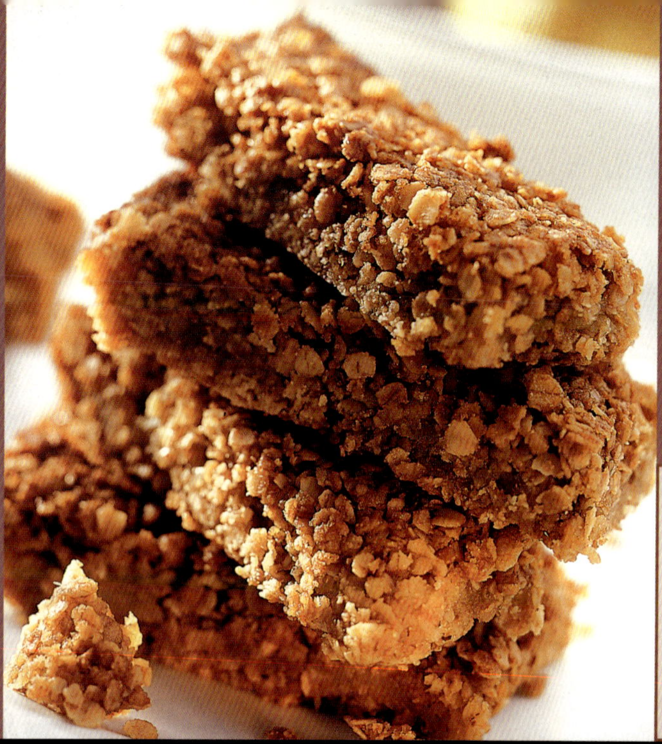

PER FLAPJACK
244 kcalories
protein 3g
carbohydrate 33g
fat 12g
saturated fat 7g
fibre 2g
added sugar 15g
salt trace

# Sweetness and light

*As you can see from the recipes in this chapter, bakes can be very good for you. The one thing that worries people, though, is the added sugar content. There are, however, ways of adding sweetness without recourse to the 'empty' calories of white sugar or the chemical uncertainties of artificial sweeteners.*

**Are there any types of sugar that are healthier than white sugar?**
*The less refined a sugar is the more nutrients it retains. For instance, white sugar has virtually nothing to offer other than simple carbohydrates (see page 36), while brown sugars do still contain traces of nutrients – generally, the darker it is in colour the more it has.*

**What are the healthier alternatives to sugar?**
*The most obvious natural sweetener is honey, which is fairly nutritious and a proven antiseptic. It is also thought by some to help purify the blood and cleanse the kidneys. As with sugar, the darker the honey, the less refined – and more whole – it is likely to be.*

*Molasses is the residue left over in the process of refining sugar and, for this reason, retains most of the nutrients stripped from the sugar. It is particularly rich in minerals like iron and calcium. Because it is so concentrated, very small quantities are required when it is used as a sweetener.*

*Fructose, the natural sugar found in fruit, is also favoured by some as it delivers about twice as much sweetness per calorie (i.e. you need half of it for the same effect). It is also thought to help reduce bad cholesterol in the blood. There are, however, dangers in using too much refined fructose, as daily intake of more than about 25g/¾oz can cause digestive problems.*

*Most nutritionists believe that refined sugars of all sorts (and even honey to a lesser extent) overtax the mechanisms that govern blood sugar levels and should be used in moderation. It is recommended that no more than 10% of your energy should come from refined/non-milk extrinsic sugars. What some nutritionists recommend is switching to natural sweeteners like those that come readily from plants without refining and much processing, such as maple syrup and date syrup.*

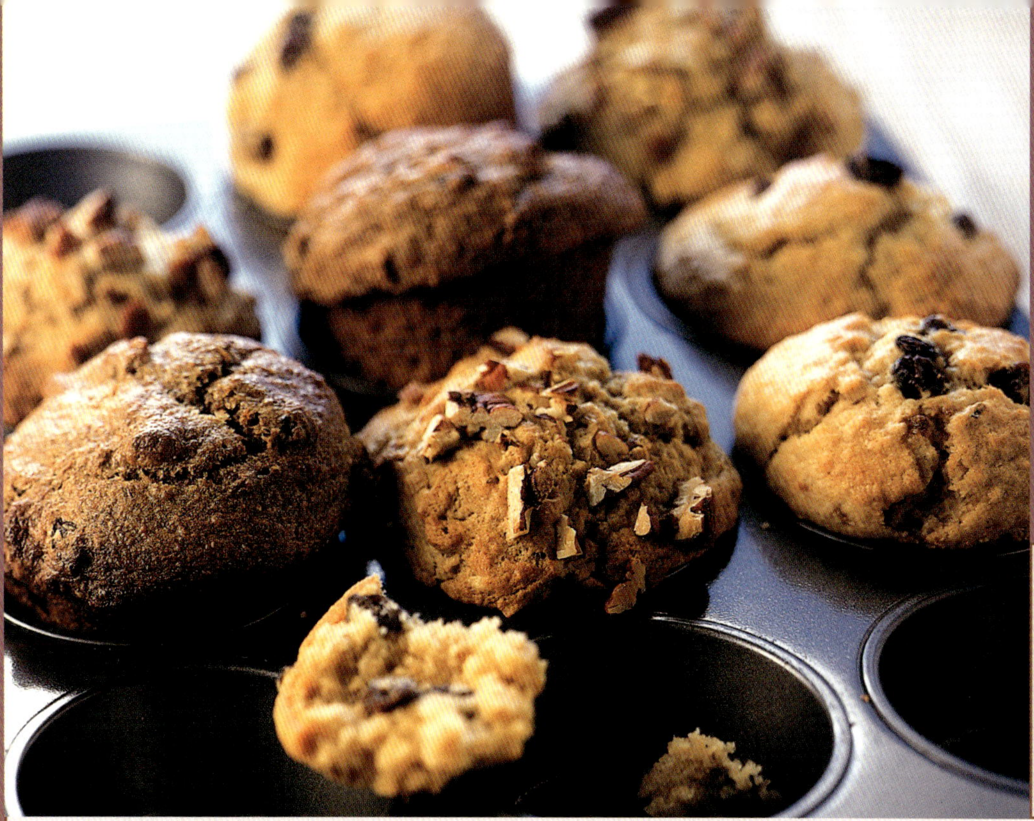

PER SERVING
283 kcalories
protein 6g
carbohydrates 44g
fat 10g
saturated fat 6g
fibre 1g
added sugar 10g
salt 0.69g

**In sweetening bakes, the strong flavours of less refined natural sweeteners, like dark brown sugar, molasses, maple syrup, etc. actually often enhance the finished effect. The large crystals of some dark sugars can also impart a delicious crunchy texture ▼**

## Date and Brown Sugar Muffins

*(above, for 6 large or 12 small), for instance, require an oven preheated to 200°C/400°F/Gas 6. Beat together 50g/2oz butter and 50g/2oz soft dark brown sugar until creamy. Beat in 2 medium eggs, one at a time, then stir in 200ml/7fl oz buttermilk.*

*Mix 100g/4oz maize meal or cornmeal, 100g/4oz rice flour and 1 rounded teaspoon baking powder in a bowl, then fold this into the other mixture. Add 50g/2oz dates, stoned and chopped. Spoon the mixture into a buttered muffin tin and bake for 25–30 minutes in the top half of the oven.*

*For banana muffins, add 1 chopped ripe banana to the batter in place of the dates. For raisin muffins, use 50g/2oz seedless raisins instead of the dates.*

## Apple Flapjacks

*(opposite for 16) require an oven preheated to 180°C/350°F/Gas 4 and a buttered tin about 17x30cm/6½x12in and 4cm/1½ in deep. Put 225g/8oz butter, 225g/8oz light muscovado sugar and 2 tablespoons golden syrup in a pan and heat gently, stirring occasionally, until the butter has melted. Don't allow the mixture to get too hot or the sugar will burn. Stir in 350g/12oz porridge oats and 1 teaspoon ground cinnamon. Remove from the heat and set aside.*

*Peel, quarter and core 2 eating apples, such as Cox's or Braeburns, then chop them into small pieces. Put in a separate pan with 2 tablespoons of cold water. Cover with a lid and cook over a medium heat for 5 minutes until the apples are soft. Drain well and set aside.*

*Press half the oat mixture into the tin, then spread the apples over the top. Spoon over the remaining oat mixture. Use a metal spoon to smooth the top (the mixture sticks to a wooden one) and press the mixture firmly into the tin. Bake on the middle shelf of the oven for 35–40 minutes until the top is golden and feels firm to the touch.*

*Leave to cool in the tin for 5 minutes then, while still warm, cut into 4 lengthwise and across to make 16 bars. Leave in the tin until cold. (Don't remove them while they're still warm or the mixture will be soft and they'll break up.) The flapjacks will keep for 3–4 days in an airtight tin.*

# Fruity Bran Muffins

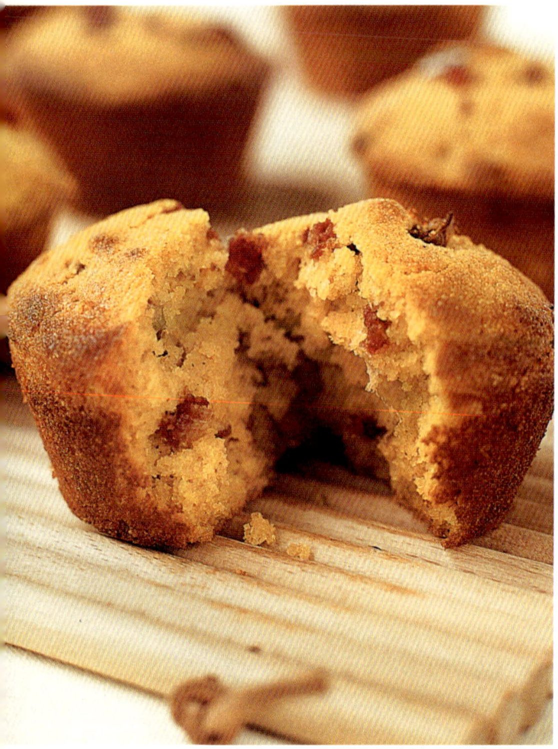

**MAKES** 16
**PREPARATION** 15 minutes
**COOKING** 15–20 minutes

50g/2oz natural bran
350g/12oz plain flour
2½ tsp bicarbonate of soda
½ tsp salt
2 eggs, beaten
150g/5oz light muscovado sugar
125ml/4fl oz vegetable oil
2 tbsp black treacle
450ml/¾ pint buttermilk
85g/3oz raisins
85g/3oz pitted dates, chopped
150g/5oz All-bran cereal
butter, for greasing

**PER MUFFIN**
**251 kcalories • protein 6g • carbohydrate 40g fat 9g • saturated fat 1g • fibre 4g added sugar 12g • salt 1g**

1 Put the natural bran in a large bowl, pour over 250ml/9fl oz boiling water, stir and allow to stand while you prepare the batter. In a second bowl, mix the flour, bicarbonate and salt.
2 In a third bowl, mix together the eggs, sugar, oil and treacle. Stir the buttermilk, raisins and dates into the bran mixture, then stir in the egg mixture. Stir in the All-bran and the flour mixture, but don't overmix. Use immediately or spoon into a plastic container with a tight-filling lid and chill for up to 3 days.
3 Preheat the oven to 200°C/400°F/Gas 6. Butter as many muffin tin holes as you want and spoon in the mixture to fill generously. Bake for 15 minutes, until risen and firm. Allow to cool on a wire rack.

# Double Chocolate Layer Cake

**PER SERVING**
**362 kcalories**
**protein 7g**
**carbohydrate 64g**
**fat 10g**
**saturated fat 6g**
**fibre 2g**
**added sugar 45g**
**salt 0.83g**

**SERVES** 12
**PREPARATION** about 1 hour, plus overnight chilling and cooling
**COOKING** 40 minutes

clean-tasting vegetable oil, for greasing
200g/7oz plus 2 tbsp plain flour
50g/2oz cocoa powder
½ tsp baking powder
½ tsp bicarbonate of soda
½ tsp salt
1 egg, plus whites of 2 more eggs
1 tbsp instant espresso or coffee powder
1½ tbsp hot water
1 tsp vanilla extract
4 tbsp buttermilk or plain yogurt
75g/3oz unsalted butter, softened
275g/9oz caster sugar
fine chocolate shavings, to decorate

**for the rich chocolate frosting**
200g/7oz caster sugar
100g/4oz cocoa powder
300ml/½ pint skimmed milk
1 tsp vanilla extract
50g/2oz milk chocolate, finely chopped

1 The day before, make frosting: put sugar and cocoa in a heavy pan with enough milk to make a smooth paste. Stir in rest over moderate heat until boiling. Boil gently for 3 minutes, stirring constantly. Off heat, stir in vanilla and chocolate until melted. Cover with greaseproof paper. Chill.
2 Next day, preheat the oven to 180°C/350°F/Gas 4, lightly oil the sides of a 20cm/8in round, 7.5cm/3in deep cake tin and line the base with greaseproof paper.
3 Sift together flour, cocoa, baking powder, bicarbonate and salt. Whisk together whole egg and whites. Dissolve coffee in hot water, then stir in vanilla and buttermilk. Beat butter until very soft. Slowly beat in sugar for 3 minutes until light and crumbly. Gradually beat in eggs for 2–3 minutes (it may look curdled). Beat in ⅓ of flour mixture, then gradually beat in ½ buttermilk. Follow with ½ remaining flour, then rest of buttermilk. Stir in remaining flour.
4 Spoon into tin and level. Bake for 40 minutes or until a skewer pushed in comes out clean. Leave in tin for 5 minutes, transfer to a rack and peel away paper. Cool.
5 Cut into 3 thin layers and sandwich with a little frosting. Spread a thin layer over top and sides. Chill for 20 minutes.
6 Spread remaining frosting over and dot with shavings.

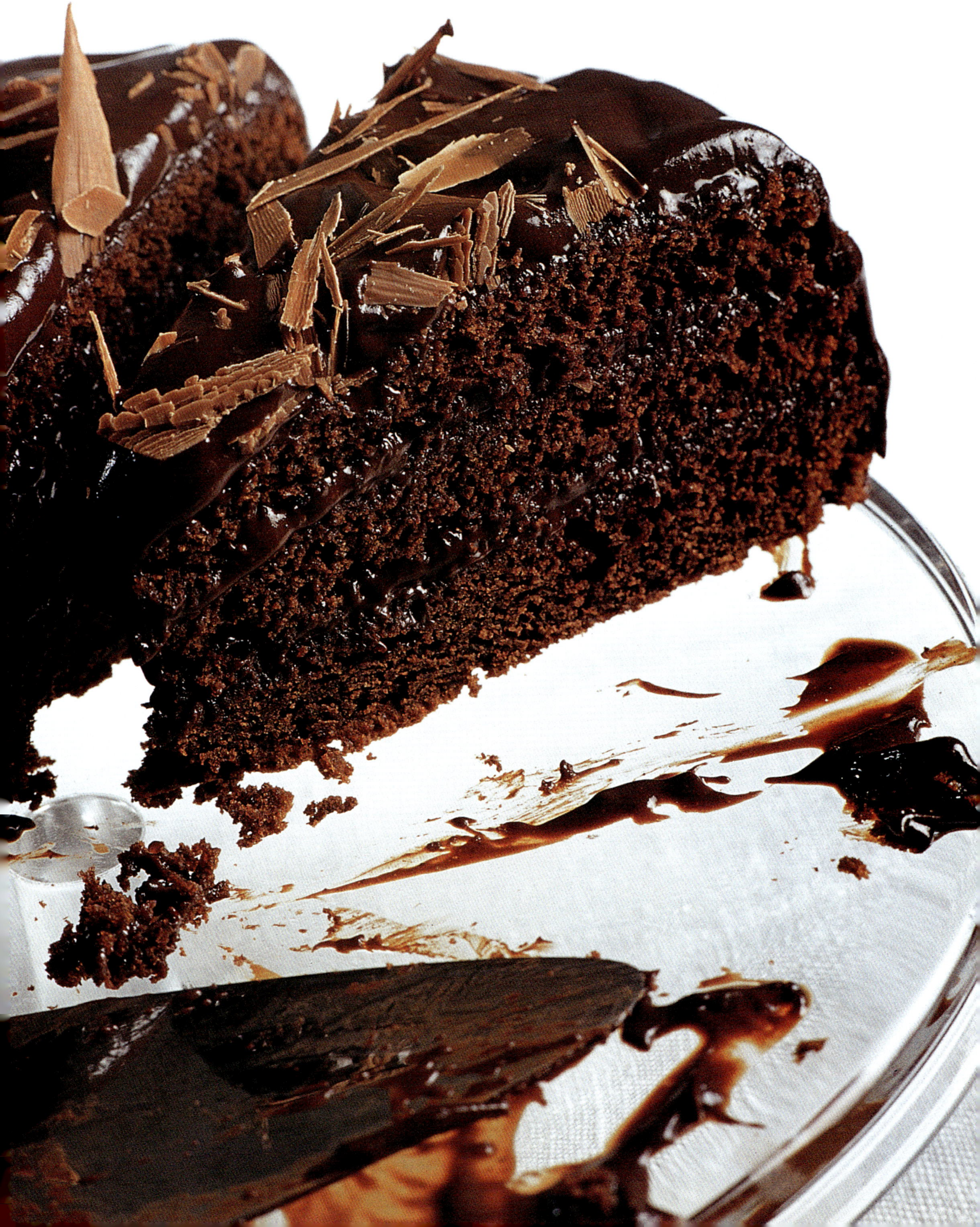

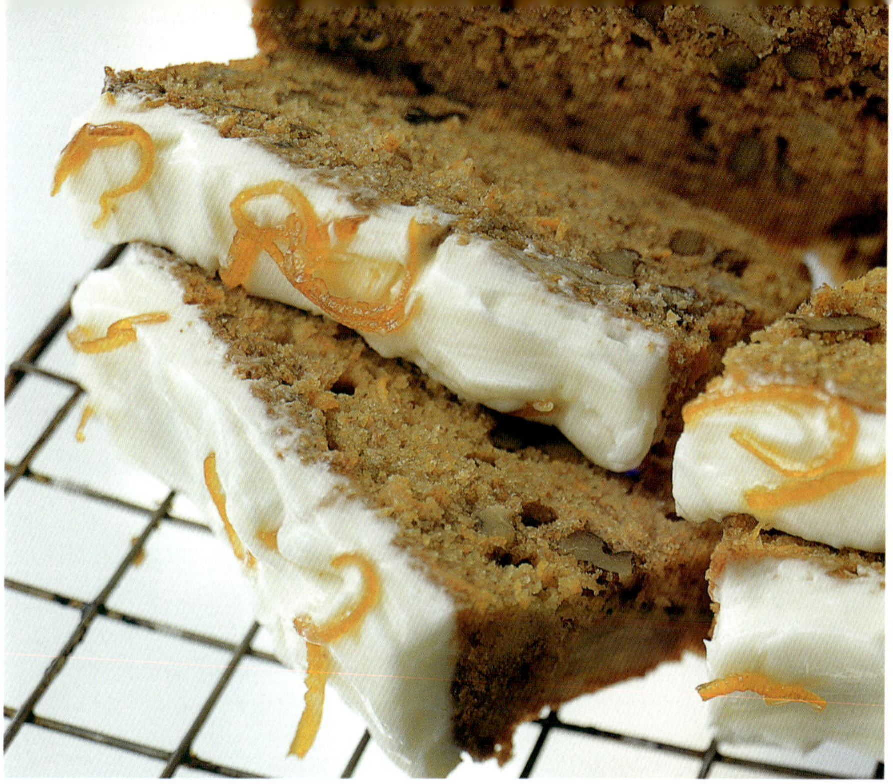

# Orange Frosted Carrot Cake

**PER SLICE (28)**
**205 kcalories**
**protein 4g**
**carbohydrate 24g**
**fat 11g**
**saturated fat 1g**
**fibre 1g**
**added sugar 13g**
**salt 0.09g**

**CUTS** into 14 slices (or 28 small ones)
**PREPARATION** 25 minutes
**COOKING** $1^{1}/_{4}$–$1^{1}/_{2}$ hours

200ml/7fl oz sunflower oil, plus more for greasing
10 cardamom pods
175g/6oz self-raising flour
175g/6oz wholemeal self-raising flour
175g/6oz light muscovado sugar
1 tsp ground cinnamon
4 eggs
200g/7oz (about 3) coarsely grated carrots
finely grated zest and juice of 1 orange
100g/4oz walnut pieces
1 medium banana, mashed

**for the crystallized orange rind**
1 orange
85g/3oz caster sugar

**for the cream cheese icing**
200g/7 oz packet of soft cheese, like Philadelphia, at room temperature
100g/4oz icing sugar

1 Preheat the oven to 180°C/350°F/Gas 4. Grease a 19cm/$7^{1}/_{2}$in square, 7.5cm/3in deep cake tin and line the base with baking parchment or greaseproof paper. Cut the cardamom pods in half and remove the seeds. Discard the pods and grind the seeds to a powder in a mortar with a pestle (or put them in a cup and use the back of a spoon). Put them in a large bowl and mix with the flours, sugar and cinnamon.
2 In a separate bowl, whisk the eggs and the 200ml/7fl oz oil with a balloon whisk until smooth. Use a large fork to stir into the flour with the carrots, orange zest and juice, walnuts and banana. Stir well (it will look like a thick batter).
3 Pour the mixture into the prepared tin and bake for $1^{1}/_{4}$–$1^{1}/_{2}$ hours until risen and firm. Cool for 10 minutes, then remove from the tin, peel off the lining paper and cool completely.
4 Make the crystallized orange rind: peel 6 strips of rind from the orange and cut each strip into matchsticks. Heat the sugar in a small pan with 3 tablespoons cold water, stirring until the sugar has dissolved. Bring to the boil, add the orange zest and simmer for 7 minutes until softened. Remove the rind and cool on greaseproof paper.
5 Make the icing: put the soft cheese in a bowl and whisk with an electric hand-whisk to soften it. Add the icing sugar a tablespoon at a time, whisking until smooth.
6 Spread the icing on the cake, swirling with a palette knife. Sprinkle over the crystallized orange rind and serve cut into slices.

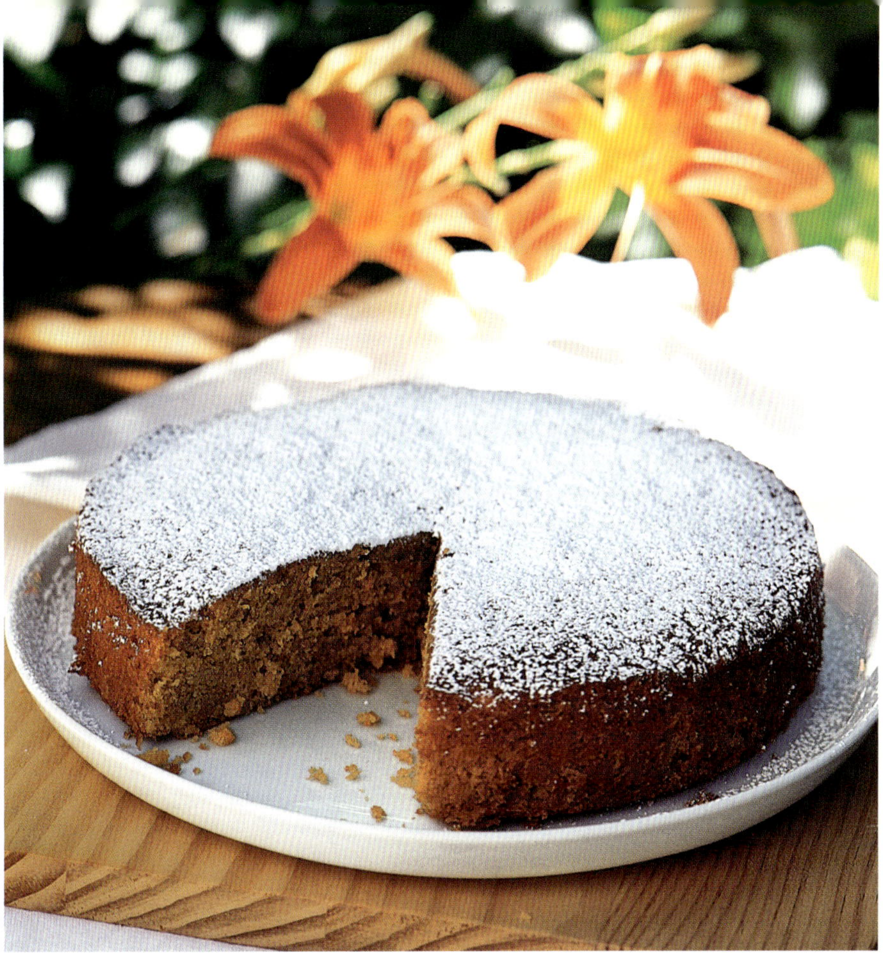

# Orange and Almond Cake

**PER SLICE**
**266 kcalories**
**protein 4g**
**carbohydrates 29g**
**fat 16g**
**saturated fat 8g**
**fibre 1g**
**added sugar 16g**
**salt 0.61g**

**This bittersweet cake is made in a most unconventional way using a puréed whole orange – the result is lovely and keeps for a week in a tin.**

CUTS into 12 slices
PREPARATION 15–20 minutes
COOKING time 25–30 minutes

1 medium orange, about 175g/6oz
175g/6oz butter, softened
175g/6oz light muscovado sugar
3 eggs
175g/6oz self-raising flour
1/2 tsp bicarbonate of soda
50g/2oz ground almonds
icing sugar, for dredging

1 Preheat the oven to 190°C/375°F/Gas 5 and grease a 23cm/9in round 5cm/2in deep cake tin, then line the base with baking parchment or greaseproof paper. Cut the whole orange – skin, pith, flesh, the lot – into pieces. Remove any pips, then whiz the orange in a food processor to a finely chopped purée.
2 Tip the butter, sugar, eggs, flour, bicarbonate of soda and almonds into the processor with the orange purée and blend for 10 seconds, until smooth. Pour into the prepared tin and smooth the top.
3 Bake for 25–30 minutes, until the cake is risen and brown. Allow to cool in the tin for 5 minutes, then turn out on to a wire rack.
4 Dredge thickly with icing sugar before serving.

# Apple Cake

**PER SERVING**
377 kcalories
protein 6g
carbohydrate 49g
fat 19g
saturated fat 8g
fibre 3g
added sugar 15g
salt 0.61g

**SERVES** 12
**PREPARATION** 15 minutes
**COOKING** 1 hour

175g/6oz butter, plus extra for greasing
3 eggs
350g/12oz self-raising flour
2 tsp ground cinnamon
175g/6oz light muscovado sugar
3 medium eating apples, such as Cox's, unpeeled but cored; 2 cut into bite-sized chunks and 1 thinly sliced
100g/4oz dates, halved and stoned
100g/4oz blanched hazelnuts, roughly chopped
3 tbsp apricot compote

1 Preheat the oven to 180°C/350°F/Gas 4 and lightly butter a 20cm/8in loose-based or spring-form cake tin, then line the base with a buttered circle of baking parchment.
2 Put the butter in a small bowl in the microwave on High for 30 seconds to 1 minute, until it has melted (or set over hot water in a small pan). Allow to cool for 5 minutes. Crack the eggs into the butter and beat well with a fork.
3 Put the flour into a bowl with the cinnamon and the sugar. Mix well until the sugar is distributed evenly.
4 Stir apple chunks into flour, together with dates and half the hazelnuts. Mix together well with a large spoon.
5 Pour egg and butter mix into flour mixture and gently stir together with a large spoon, making sure flour is completely mixed in. Spoon mixture into the prepared tin. Smooth top using a palette knife or flat-bladed table knife.
6 Arrange apple slices on top. Sprinkle over remaining nuts and bake for 50–60 minutes until cooked and risen. Check by pushing a skewer into the centre – it should come out clean. Let cool in the tin for 5 minutes.
7 Remove cake from tin, peel off paper and transfer to a rack. While still warm, heat the apricot compote in a small pan until it just begins to bubble. Brush the warm compote over the top of the cake then allow to cool completely before cutting. Eat within 3 days.

# Apple and Cinnamon Cake

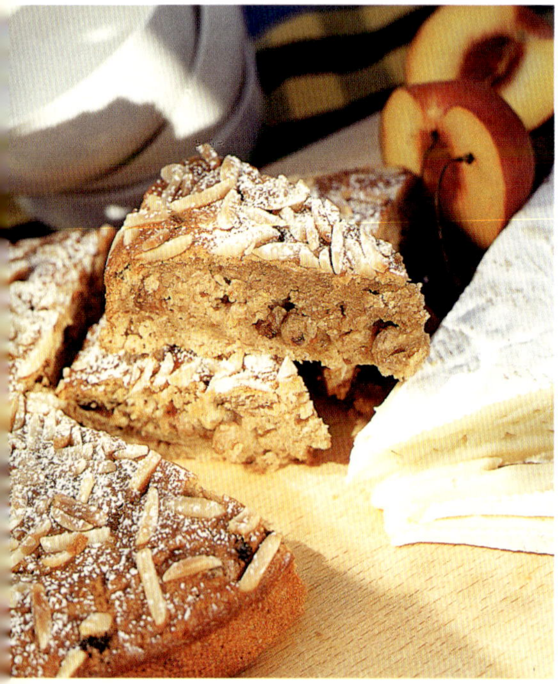

**CUTS** into 8–10 slices
**PREPARATION** 20 minutes
**COOKING** 40–45 minutes

250g/9oz self-raising flour
1 tsp ground cinnamon
1 tsp baking powder
100g/4oz light muscovado sugar
175g/6oz sultanas or raisins
125ml/4fl oz sunflower oil
2 eggs, beaten
125ml/4fl oz apple juice
2 dessert apples (unpeeled), grated
30g/1oz slivered or flaked almonds
icing sugar, for dusting

**PER SERVING**
342 kcalories • protein 6g • carbohydrate 46g
fat 16g • saturated fat 2g • fibre 2g
added sugar 10g • salt 0.46g

1 Preheat the oven to 180°C/350°F/Gas 4. Line a 23cm/9in round, 5cm/2in deep cake tin with baking paper. Sift the flour into a bowl with the cinnamon and baking powder, then stir in the sugar and sultanas or raisins. Make a well in the centre and stir in the oil, eggs, apple juice and grated apple until well mixed.
2 Pour the mixture into the tin, scatter with almonds, then bake for 40–45 minutes until firm in the centre or a skewer inserted into the middle comes out clean. Leave to cool in the tin for about 5 minutes, then turn out and allow to cool completely on a wire rack.
3 Dust with icing sugar to serve.

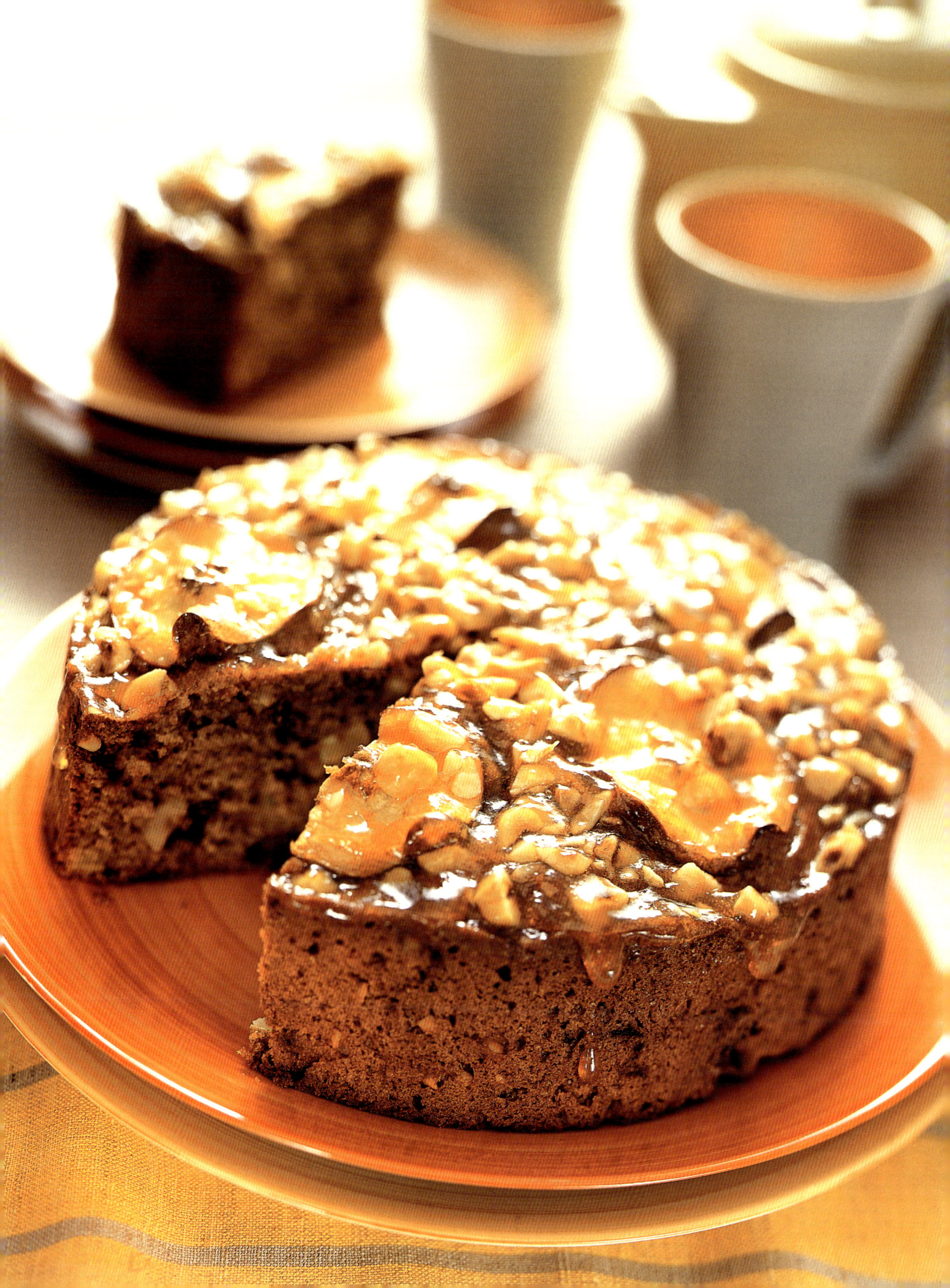

# Acknowledgements

Features and most recipe introductions: Lewis Esson

Nutritional Consultant: Dr Wendy Doyle

## Recipes by

### Sue Ashworth
Lemon and herb chicken in a pot p45, Rösti chicken breasts with red cabbage p87, New vegetables à la Grecque p102, Pistachio plums with orange syrup p117

### Annie Bell
Warm potato, mussel and squid salad p92

### Mary Cadogan
Leafy artichoke and crisp prosciutto salad p26, Smoked trout and dill blinis p30, Gravadlax p33, Quick chicken satay p46, Thai chicken and coconut curry p46, Cod and tomato stew p59, Salmon with spring onions and sizzled garlic p89, Cod with pesto and potato slices p90, Cod and prawn casserole with pesto toasts p91

### Mary Cadogan and Vicky Musselman
Salmon, cannellini and lemon crumb stew p88

### Robert Carrier
Seven-vegetable couscous p105

### Michael Cox
Date and brown sugar muffins p133, taken from his book *Great Healthy Food Gluten-free* (Carroll & Brown)

### Shona Crawford Poole
Cream of mushroom soup p25, Wild mushroom risotto p40

### Emma Crowhurst
Pork tenderloin with herb crust and tomato dressing p68

### Lewis Esson
Sensational smoothies p15, Chillied trout with Chinese leaves p79

### Silvana Franco
Balsamic onion and goats' cheese salad p28, Spicy pepper penne p56, Glazed duck with pasta ribbons p85, Filo trout tartlets with broccoli stir-fry p92, Frozen redcurrant and ginger crush p115, Mango meringue fool p120, Lemon sponge drops p122

### Susanna Gelmetti
Courgette and saffron risotto p40

### The Good Food Team
Eggs from the Med p11, Potato and red pepper tortilla p11, Ratatouille omelette p19, Smoked haddock and leek risotto p20, Aubergine and mozzarella stacks p26, Warm mackerel and beetroot salad p29, Warm potato and tuna salad with pesto dressing p39, Creamy broccoli and mushroom pasta p39, Chicken with apples and cider p45, Braised winter chicken and vegetables p49, Mediterranean chicken pasta p49, Ratatouille meatballs p51, Meal-in-a-bowl noodle soup p52, Spinach and feta pizza pie p53, Spaghetti Genovese p54, Summer spaghetti with tomato and brie p55, Double cheese and tuna pasta p56, Trout with warm potato salad p59, Quick fish pie p60, Cod fillets with pan-fried cabbage p61, Rosemary lamb kebabs with runner bean spaghetti pp62-3, Turkey and sweet potato gratin p69, Barbecued coriander chicken with guacamole salsa p71, Chinese chicken stir-fry p71, Moroccan chicken and chickpeas p74, Chicken with a red pepper and parsley crust p75, Lemon cod with spicy chickpeas p78, Venison with herbed pumpkin wedges p83, Pan-fried beef with garlic, rosemary and balsamic vinegar p83, Panzanella p99, Roasted vegetable rice p104, Thai vegetable curry p108, Roasted roots with Indian spices p109, Gin and tonic granita p113, Summer fruits ice yoghurt p114, Apricot flapjack crumble p117, Fried rum bananas p118

### Sophie Grigson
Chicken, fennel and tomato ragout p73

### Mary Gwynn
Spiced vegetable pancake stack p107

### Ainsley Harriott
Spice'n'sizzle prawns on black-eyed bean salsa p32

### Marie José Sevilla
Seafood pasta p95

### Alice Medrich
Chocolate marble cheesecake p125, Chocolate cookies p131, Double chocolate layer cake p134, all from her book *Chocolate and the Art of Low-fat Desserts* (Warner Books), copyright Alice Medrich 1994. By permission of Little, Brown & Company (Inc.)

### Kate Moseley
Turkey and mushroom fusilli p51

### Orlando Murrin
Parsnip pancakes with soy dipping sauce p12, Sweetcorn fritters p12, Linguine with watercress sauce p37, Chicken with 40 cloves of garlic p74, Beetroot and chickpea salad p99, Baked buttery squash p106

### Vicky Musselman
Salmon stir-fry with wilted leaves p77, Apple flapjacks p133, Orange frosted carrot cake p146, Orange and almond cake p137, Apple cake p138

### Angela Nilsen
Banana and apricot compote p17, Pancakes with honey and ricotta p17, Oriental prawn tagliatelle salad p34, Roasted pepper and prosciutto spaghetti salad p34, Mustard and pepper crusted lamb with new potatoes p65, Spicy beef with pumpkin and corn p66, Oriental stir-fried lamb with mushrooms p66, Paper-wrapped salmon with orange butter, fennel and mushrooms p77, Thai prawns en papillote with coconut milk p95, 30-minute summer pudding p126, Chunky chocolate nut flapjacks p131, Fruity bran muffins p134, Apple and cinnamon cake p138

### Angela Nilsen and Jenny White
Margarita chilli sorbet p113

### Bridget Sargeson
Red cabbage with prunes p101, Tian of root vegetables p102

### Linda Tubby
Garlic lemon spinach p101

### Phil Vickery
Salad of braised winter vegetables with toasted hazelnut dressing p24

### Lesley Waters
Spiced root veg with mackerel

and fried eggs p18, Pancakes with hot passion fruit sauce p126

### Jenny White
Chicken and pumpkin Cajun gumbo p84, Fragrant rosé peaches p121, Cinnamon cake and caramelized pineapple with rum sauce p123

### Anne Willan
Hot toddy chicken breasts p72, Roast brandy plums with ginger p119

### Lorna Wing
Watermelon, prawn and cucumber salad p30

### Jean Wright
Griddled polenta with porcini p21

## Photographers

### Chris Alack
Chinese chicken stir-fry p71

### Marie-Louise Avery
Turkey and mushroom fusilli p51, Seafood pasta p95

### Jean Cazals
Smoked haddock and leek risotto p20, Griddled polenta with porcini p21. Smoked trout and dill blinis p31, Spaghetti with courgettes p37, Courgette and saffron risotto p40, Mustard and pepper crusted lamb with new potatoes p64, Oriental stir-fried lamb with mushrooms p67, Paper-wrapped salmon with orange butter, fennel and mushrooms p76, Venison with herbed pumpkin wedges pp80-1, Pan-fried beef with garlic, rosemary and balsamic vinegar p82, Salmon, cannellini and lemon crumb stew p88, Salmon with spring onions and sizzled garlic p89, Thai prawns en papillote with coconut milk p94, Panzanella p98, Roasted roots with Indian spices p109, Margarita chilli sorbet pp110-1, Pancakes with hot passion fruit sauce p127

### Gus Filgate
Seven-vegetable couscous p105

### Ian Garlick
Date and brown sugar muffins p133

### Sandra Lane
Garlic lemon spinach p101

### William Lingwood
Pancakes with honey and ricotta p17

### David Munns
Sweetcorn fritters p13, Watermelon, prawn and cucumber salad p30, Chillied trout with Chinese leaves p79, Beetroot and chickpea salad pp96-7, Baked buttery squash p107, Apple cake p139

### Nick Pope
Leafy artichoke and crisp prosciutto salad p27

### William Reavell
Balsamic onion and goats' cheese salad p28, Glazed duck with pasta ribbons p85, Lemon sponge drops p122

### Diane Seed
Spaghetti with courgettes p37

### Simon Smith
Linguine with watercress sauce p36, Salmon stir-fry with wilted leaves p77

### Roger Stowell
Eggs from the Med pp8-9, Potato and red pepper tortilla p10, Sensational smoothies p14, Ratatouille omelette p19, Warm mackerel and beetroot salad p29, Warm potato and tuna salad with pesto dressing p38, Chicken with apples and cider p44, Braised winter chicken and vegetables p48, Mediterranean chicken pasta p49, Ratatouille meatballs p50, Meal-in-a-bowl noodle soup p52, Spinach and feta pizza pie p53, Spaghetti Genovese p54, Summer spaghetti with tomato and brie p55, Double cheese and tuna pasta p56, Trout with warm potato salad p59, Quick fish pie p60, Cod fillets with pan-fried cabbage p61, Rosemary lamb kebabs with runner bean spaghetti pp62-3, Turkey and sweet potato gratin p69, Barbecued coriander chicken with guacamole salsa p70, Chicken with a red pepper and parsley crust p75, Lemon cod with spicy chickpeas p78, Roasted vegetable rice p104, Summer fruits ice yoghurt p114, Apricot flapjack crumble p117, Fried rum bananas p118, Apple flapjacks p132, Orange and almond cake p137

### Sam Stowell
Gin and tonic granita p112, Frozen redcurrant and ginger crush p115, Cinnamon cake and caramelized pineapple with rum sauce p123

### Martin Thompson
Gravadlax p33, Spicy pepper penne p57, Pork tenderloin with herb crust and tomato dressing p68, Cod and prawn casserole with pesto toasts p91

### Ian Wallace
30-minute summer pudding p126

### Philip Webb
Spiced root veg with mackerel and fried eggs p18, Salad of braised winter vegetables with toasted hazelnut dressing p22-3, Cream of mushroom soup p25, Aubergine and mozzarella stacks p26, Oriental prawn tagliatelle salad p34, Roasted pepper and prosciutto spaghetti salad p35, Wild mushroom risotto p41, Lemon and herb chicken in a pot pp42-3, Hot toddy chicken breasts p72, Chicken, fennel and tomato ragout p73, Chicken and pumpkin Cajun gumbo p84, Rösti chicken breasts with red cabbage p86, Filo trout tartlets with broccoli stir-fry p92, Warm potato, mussel and squid salad p93, Red cabbage with prunes p100, Tian of root vegetables p103, Pistachio plums with orange syrup p116, Roast brandy plums with ginger p119, Mango meringue fool p120, Fragrant rosé peaches p121, Chunky chocolate nut flapjacks pp128-9, Fruity bran muffins p134, Orange frosted carrot cake p136

### Simon Wheeler
Banana and apricot compote p16, Thai chicken and coconut curry p46, Quick chicken satay p47, Cod and tomato stew p58, Cod with pesto and potato slices p90, Chocolate marble cheesecake p124, Chocolate cookies p130, Double chocolate layer cake p135, Apple and cinnamon cake p138

### Jon Whitaker
Parsnip pancakes with soy dipping sauce p12

### Geoff Wilkinson
Spice'n'sizzle prawns on black-eyed bean salsa p32, Spicy beef with pumpkin and corn p66, Thai vegetable curry p108

Whilst every effort has been made to trace and acknowledge all copyright holders, we would like to apologize should there be any errors or omissions.

# Index